Quantum Healing

Discover The Power Of Self-healing
And Laws Of Quantum

(Passing Through The Eye Of The Needle Into Self-actualization)

Jimmy Ruiz

Published By **Bella Frost**

Jimmy Ruiz

All Rights Reserved

Quantum Healing: Discover The Power Of Self-healing And Laws Of Quantum (Passing Through The Eye Of The Needle Into Self-actualization)

ISBN 978-1-77485-675-8

No part of this guidebook shall be reproduced in any form without permission in writing from the publisher except in the case of brief quotations embodied in critical articles or reviews.

Legal & Disclaimer

The information contained in this ebook is not designed to replace or take the place of any form of medicine or professional medical advice. The information in this ebook has been provided for educational & entertainment purposes only.

The information contained in this book has been compiled from sources deemed reliable, and it is accurate to the best of the Author's knowledge; however, the Author cannot guarantee its accuracy and validity and cannot be held liable for any errors or omissions. Changes are periodically made to this book. You must consult your doctor or get professional medical advice before using any of the suggested remedies, techniques, or information in this book.

Upon using the information contained in this book, you agree to hold harmless the Author from and against any damages, costs, and expenses, including any legal fees potentially resulting from the application of any of the information provided by this guide. This disclaimer applies to any damages or injury caused by the use and application, whether directly or indirectly, of any advice or information presented, whether for breach of contract, tort, negligence, personal injury, criminal intent, or under any other cause of action.

You agree to accept all risks of using the information presented inside this book. You need to consult a professional medical practitioner in order to ensure you are both able and healthy enough to participate in this program.

TABLE OF CONTENTS

Chapter 1: Introduction 1

Chapter 2: Dreams That Comes True 10

Chapter 3: The Early Experiences Of Healing 20

Chapter 4: Healing Principles..........26

Chapter 5: A Plan To Be Healed 45

Chapter 6: The Role Of Love In Healing 51

Chapter 7: The Process Of Awareness Is The First Step To Healing.............57

Chapter 8: Zero Point Of Stillness ...64

Chapter 9: Listening Can Be Therapeutic 79

Chapter 10: Vata, Pitta & Kapha.....88

Chapter 11: Health And Emotions 103

Chapter 12: The Overview Of 3 Methods 110

Chapter 13: Guidelines Prior To When We Begin 115

Chapter 14: T1 - Heart Energy Healing 132

Chapter 15: Basic Techniques 151

Chapter 16: Synchronizing 173

Chapter 1: Introduction

Instantly heal? Yes ! It's true. You'll be able to heal yourself and others, and this will happen almost instantly.

If you know the fundamental aspects of how healing happens and adhere to the easy instructions by this text, you'll be able to heal patients in a matter of minutes having read this book, in only 7 hours of care. According to my experience healing more than 600 people suffering from various ailments healing begins with a single click, the symptoms of which are noticed immediately by the healer and are also felt by the patient being treated.

In the past three years I had the pleasure of using these methods of healing on patients who are suffering from health issues like knee back pain, pain in the knee, frozen shoulder, headaches Migraine, Digestive disorders Constipation Acidity, Gastritis, Indigestion, Ear Ache, Throat Pain, Menstrual Cramps, Irregular Menstrual cycle, tooth pain and skin problems Cervical spondylitis Slipped Disc Varicose Veins, Twisted limbs Sprains, Swellings, Injuries and wounds, fractures, Heel Spur and Sinus-related issues and Stomach Ache Liver disorders Psoriasis, IBS, swollen fingers because of arthritis, Sciatica problems, Vertigo Thyroid problems and even early stages of Cancer.

Within 7 to 10 minutes of treatment, over 50 percent of the cases treated immediately. 30 percent of patients reported complete relief within the next 12-to-18 hours. 10 % required 1 or 2 sessions to experience full relief. In the remaining 10% of cases healing didn't happen as they expectedit to, but in a different part of their life which was more crucial in the larger picture that they hadn't even mentioned to me.

I have noticed that the individual's soul or spirit energy, as well as the life force that is universal determines the priority and the order in which healing can occur on a Physical Level (Health and Wealth, Possessions, etc.) as well as an emotional level (Love and Relationship) or on a spiritual level (Peace and awakening)

The techniques are extremely efficient and effective and can provide the instant results. the shortest healing time that lasts between 5 and seven minutes. This is much faster than any other traditional method of treatment. Other approaches like Surgery, Allopathy, Ayurveda, Homeopathy, Physiotherapy etc. will take a few hours or weeks to achieve the desired outcomes.

Conventional medicine usually addresses the symptoms, but it isn't the primary source of the problem. The issue is then recurred after a time. Furthermore, the unfavorable unwanted side effects associated with traditional medicines/drugs must be considered as component of treatment.

The methods for healing that I have described in this book don't have any negative consequences. They will only benefit but it will not cause harm to the person who is being healed as well as the person who is healing. I've heard there are various alternative healing methodsthat healers must be extremely vigilant, as the condition of the person who is being healed could be passed on to the healer, and this could be a source of concern for the healer. The techniques I have described here don't face this issue, as the healer isn't doing the healing. It is the body that heals person who is being treated, as well as the universe work together to perform the healing. The healer must be 'nothing'. I've explained in the book exactly what "Doing Nothing" means and how it can bring about healing in a matter of minutes.

In all other treatments In all other treatments, it's the expertise of the physician, or the inbuilt intelligence of the medication, that creates the final result. The doctor chooses the type of treatment dose and frequency, as well as the location where to administer it, and for the length of time. When any of the above goes wrong, then it may cause problems with regards to negative side consequences. When we perform healing with the methods I have discussed the universal energy source with infinite intelligence is able to take over the healing process , without having to be influenced or input on the part of the practitioner. It performs whatever is needed to reach a state that is health and harmony. So there aren't any side negative effects.

These methods of healing produce resultseven without being able to identify the issue or what the reason is. We can effectively heal people even when we do not know what's wrong with them. There have been instances in which people didn't tell me about any secondary issues they were experiencing. After my healing session they reported that in addition to the main issues, these were also completely resolved and even though they didn't tell me of it. Thus, I believe it's the body's own intelligence, together with the intelligence of the universe, that's at work. It is able to discern what's not in balance, and what needs to be restored.

It's a different story in contrast to conventional medical treatments in which a correct diagnosis is crucial as well as, often, incorrect diagnosis can lead to the improper treatment, which then can cause complications. In traditional medical treatment, the doctor has to determine the cause and then only the correct approach is selected. The expertise and knowledge of the physician is crucial and without it the treatment may be completely unsuitable.

These healing methods don't require any knowledge about human biology, medicine or the way healing occurs. Even a five-year-old child can be able to successfully help other people. Any person who is of any age, background or gender can heal. It is also not related to do with religious beliefs or the belief system of God.

The healing process doesn't require the presence of our intellect or our minds. It actually requires the absence of our minds. It is possible to think, "why is our mind not necessary?". The truth is that the human body is such an intricate system, it is impossible for our mind can be aware of what's going on and how it functions. The understanding of our mind about the human body and medical science is very limited.

You may be aware that according to Ayurveda an imbalance in Vata-Pitta and Kapha causes disease and joint muscle pains or issues with the Musculoskeletal system are caused by imbalance with Vata. However, modern medicine doesn't accept this fact at all.

My observations are that in a majority of cases of musculoskeletal pain at the point I begin healing process, there is an influx of gas that is activated. In a subsequent chapter I've described how a treatment of 5 minutes caused a person to release gas continuously for about 8 hours. Then the patient was completely free of chronic neck pain and migraine. Does any doctor believe that this much gas could be trapped within our joints or in the spine? The doctor could simply prescribe medication and painkillers to alleviate the symptoms (pain) and in more severe instances, would likely suggest procedure to address the issue.

In short it is not necessary to utilize our minds or our intellect when the all-knowing universe has done its work. All we need is to use our intuition that is directed by our spiritual self and knows the universe more than our brains.

Another intriguing aspect of these healing techniques is that they can be carried out even if you are located far from the person receiving healing. Even if we're located in a different town or state, or even a different country around the globe, healing is still working. Two of the 3 techniques that are described in this book even when we're in contact with one another it is not necessary to physically touch the person healing. It's possible to do the work at an extended distance.

If this seems exciting to you, and you're wondering whether you'll be able to become a healerthen let me assure you that this is a talent that all of us have been born with. The problem is that we are not aware of this natural talent and live in a dim view of our full potential.

The book I've tried to provide 3 Powerful Healing Techniques in a simple manner.

T1- Heart Energy Healing

The T2 Listening Technique - Listening to your body

T3- Zero Point Healing

The T1 and the T2 are so easy to begin using them effectively within a matter of 10 minutes of studying the necessary steps even if you've not yet read the rest part of the text. It is recommended to read the whole book to gain an knowledge of the concepts and how to apply them, however, this is not required to heal.

Alongside the essential principles, I've explained everything you'll have to know and do when you're healing yourself or someone else. To aid you in this, and the specifics of each technique I've also shared several real-life healing experiences I've had over the last four years. This will provide you with an idea of what you will experience as you go through your healing.

I am confident that this book will teach you the ability to help people heal and when you are practicing and improve, you'll become more proficient at it. If you keep practicing these methods, new possibilities will begin to open up and you may achieve what is commonly referred to as impossible.

I urge you to join in this amazing journey to become healer. You will not only heal yourself, but also aid others in dealing with health problems they may face. I guarantee you that this will bring you tremendous joy, happiness and self-healing as well as others. I encourage you to remain open to everything that is in this book and to open your mind to the thrilling process of discovering this mysterious talent.

I can assure I can assure you that your time, effort and effort that you put into this book will prove to be among the most beneficial investment decisions of your life.

I would like to wish you the best when you begin your journey to becoming Healer ! !

***

Chapter 2: Dreams That Comes True

The year 2016 saw a vision that was in my head for quite a long time suddenly came to life. For the past year, around the conclusion of each year, I've written goals for the coming year, usually pertaining to Income, Health business, personal life. But my goals for 2016 that I wrote down in December 2015, contained an additional purpose. It was to develop spiritual awareness and the capability to heal people suffering from health problems.

Since my early school days I've always been intrigued by the possibility of healing people. However, I wasn't certain how I would go about doing this. After graduating in Mechanical engineering I joined Godrej as an engineer in Design. In the interest of healing, I started studying Reiki in 1995. However I was unable to be successful in healing with Reiki. I went on to complete the MBA in Marketing and focusing exclusively on my work. Because of my passion I entered the field of corporate training and in 2008, I launched my own training and consulting company called "Transform to Lead'. We offer leadership and behavioural skills training. The need to heal was always there within my subconscious mind.

Beginning in 2014, every now and then I'd be asking my self, "What am I here to do, and what is it I am doing to benefit humanity?". In the absence of a convincing answer is enough to disturb me. If I ever spoke about this issue with my wifeshe'd inform me that I was fortunate to work in a field that was my own choice. In some ways, my education and coaching helped people. But my own inner voice would tell me that it was something I was doing to earn to earn a living. This could not be the only reason behind my presence here on the planet. There was certainly something more significant for which I was on earth But what was it? There was no way to know. In that moment I didn't know that in 2016 I would find the answer to my question.

As a person, have always thought of my self as a mechanical, with an oil can, who has come to earth to help solve issues. I was astonished to see the way that some people (saints) are able to contact people and instantly heal them. I would think about how wonderful it would be should I have the same abilities. This thought was on my mind for some time particularly during the last quarter of the year. That's what inspired me to make that goal declaration at the close this year. It seems that once something becomes the top priority of one's life then it is the will of the Universe to help make it occur.

In 2016, my dream came to an actuality and I embarked on the path of Healing. In addition to working in area of Leadership development I also devote a significant amount of my time helping people heal. After helping over 600 people find some relief from various medical problems it has now been a lifelong goal for me and I'm thoroughly enjoying every minute of it. The training I am involved in puts me in contact with lots of people each month, and offers me a lot of opportunities to assist people. This is something I want to be able to do until I'm living on this planet.

This interesting journey started. My first experience trying to help someone heal was a huge success, and this is what motivated me to continue to this point and with lots of confidence. This is what transpired.

In August I was on my way to Gujarat to conduct a Training program. I realised that deep inside my being, I was still and in silence. My awareness was at its highest. I was completely conscious of the NOW and my thoughts had nearly disappeared. The feeling was one of bliss and joy. I was reminded that in some of the articles I read found on the web, I discovered that in an ethereal state and no-mind, one gains the capacity to heal oneself and others.

In my return journey, I began reading about different methods of healing at a quantum scale. In one article, it was said that we can help others heal by simply making a conscious decision to heal in a state that is consciousness and employing the Heart energy i.e. love to heal. My experience was that the initial condition i.e. having a healing intention in my mind was easy and that second one i.e. an awareness state of Silence' is something I was experiencing deeply at the moment. The only additional thing that had to be done was to express an emotion of affection by my heart into the suffering body of the other , and healing would occur quickly. (This can be described as the Technique T1 described in chapter 14 of the book).

It was a bit overwhelming, but I was keen to try it to determine if it actually did work. The only question was ...who should I test with it? I had this question on my mind while I drove back from Gujarat. However, I did not know that one day later the universe would offer me the chance to test it.

I got home around 5AM and decided to go to bed for a few hours. After a few hours I awoke to someone speaking loudly. The woman who works at my house as a domestic assistant was complaining of severe back pain. She was also asking my wife to take a week's vacation. The doctor who treated her had advised her she suffered from a Slipped Disc, and needed to rest completely for one week.

I walked out to the living room and began to listen to the conversations. Evidently, the intensity of the pain she was experiencing was intense that she could not sit straight. She was bent over, and one leg was hurting and making her limp. I instantly realized that this was an ideal opportunity to try to help her heal, however, I still was in a state of confusion about what to do and how healing would take place. I also knew the fact that, if I did not attempt it, I'd not be able to overcome this mess.

Then, I came to my mind, and told her I was going to test a specific treatment without touching her that could provide her with relief. I informed her that I would try for 5 minutes and then we'd check for any changes. I sat in front of her, fixed my gaze at her lower back. I came into a state of consciousness and began sending an intense, unconditional affection through my heart chakra to the lower part of her back with the intention of healing it.

After about two minutes, i considered asking her whether she felt any change. But, before I could do this, she reverted and informed me that something was moving within her back. She felt intense vibrations in her spine and was feeling like something was pulling her in the back. I was also astonished that something had actually started occurring within her body and I realized that I was most likely heading on the right track. I was just required to continue the way I was.

After another 3 minutes of therapy I requested her to stand up and see whether there had been any changes. After she stood to her delight, her pain was gone. She tried to turn her body in every direction just to make sure. She smiled on her face and informed me that the back pain was gone. There was a little pain on her leg. After that, I treated her for another 5 minutes following which the pain in her leg was gone completely. She was in a position to stand straight and walk straight without limping. I realized that I had made it through my first attempt to heal. Imagine how thrilled and exuberant I felt.

After that incident I was ecstatic to try this method on other people. I was certain that if invested my energy into this, I'd be able to improve this incredible ability more. The subsequent days, I was constantly looking for patients suffering from some or some other type of discomfort or pain I could help. It was fortunate that my job i.e. training delivery, opened up this chance for me. In the tea breaks of each program I would inform the participants about my new abilities and offer the possibility of healing anyone suffering from an disease during our lunch break or at night.

Usually, I would have at least 4-5 persons in each group who were experiencing issues like neck pain, back pain and leg pain as well as other health problems. Many times, people would request me to instruct them on techniques. So, after my presentation lasting between 1 and 1.5 hours, I taught participants ways to treat themselves as well as other people. This was repeated for the subsequent sessions, and continues to be still being taught to this day.

The most satisfying part was that 80-90 percent of the patients I treated on day one of the program would inform me on the following day that they were completely healed. This greatly increased my confidence to try this treatment method for other ailments. It allowed me to gain invaluable experience working with different health issues and also gave me insight on the different ways people react to this method of treatment.

As a result I also began to experiment using two additional healing methods (T2 and T3 mentioned within this publication). Within a short time following this, I experienced more than 250 healing experiences in the following four years I experienced more than 600 experiences of healing. Each one provided me with a new understanding of the power of healing.

I'd read somewhere that coins made of metal or water are able to contain healing energy. So , once I tried placing my intention to heal into a glass and the energy of healing and asked a lady who had been seeking medical treatment, to consume it. When she consumed the drink, she experienced an energy shift in her body. Eventually, her issue was solved. One time, when my house maid was suffering from pain, I offered her a small piece of coin I had placed my healing consciousness into. And as I asked her place the coin on the body of her, she began experiencing vibrations within her body, and the pain went away. These experiences opened the door to a variety of possibilities for experimenting with healing.

The most interesting aspect was that I had absolutely nothing about how healing was occurring. The more I avoided letting my brain and mind away from my healing, more rapid was the result. It was all I needed to do was to express the awareness of my heart, Love, and intent and the universe would take care of the rest.

I'm not a medical professional and I have no knowledge about the insides of the body and how it functions. I've completely relied on the tools that I have learned, my universal intelligence and intuition to help me. It's clear that I am not the one who does the healing, rather there is a powerful force that knows precisely what's wrong, and how to rectify it quickly. What it basically meant was that I was free of the obligation of creating healing for other people.

Since 2016, I've been offering healing sessions to people to offer a service to humanity, and without charging any cost. I always inform people upfront that they have to be open to what the universe is requesting to bring about and I am unable to assure any healing. This also helps keep their expectations in check. My experience is that the majority of patients come back to their homes with amazing experiences and healing.

***

***

Chapter 3: The Early Experiences Of Healing

The reason I am sharing few of my experiences with healing is to inspire you to learn more about the healing techniques and the speed at which they can be used. In addition, once you understand that the healings took place within the first one to 2 months following my began this process, it will give the confidence that you will get the same results, in a matter of minutes.

I have provided the following three experiences for healing. In the first I utilized Technique (T1) in which I emitted the love energy emanating from me to the person's neck, and it healing in a matter of only a few minutes. In the second I utilized Technique (T2) In this technique, I was able to listen for the message of a hand using my palms and healing occurred naturally to it. In the third I've employed Technique (T3) i.e. Zero Point awareness and entrainment to treat frozen shoulders instantly.

1. Healing Experience (Heart Energy Healing)

One of my clients called me by telephone one day, and told me the company he worked for was Hindustan Petroleum Corporation Limited. A friend of his, who been to my training course was able to inform him of the way I heal. He was suffering from extreme neck pain and needed my help in removing that. Because he was so far from me, I informed me I'd try to help him with remote therapy i.e. distant healing.

I chose to utilize Heart Energy healing, in which one must send the love energy from their heart into the part of their body that requires healing. This method of healing works best when it is done face-to-face with another person, or at a distance with an image or even one's imagination.

I requested him to send me a picture with his neck clearly visible. Then, I conducted five minutes of healing by transmitting the energy of love of my heart the neck as shown in the photo, with the intention of healing it. The next day, I received his message that his pain had decreased by nearly 70 percent. I followed up with another remote healing session, following which he was completely free from discomfort.

Healing Experience 2. (Listening to body signals)

This was a healing experience for an amputee who suffered from extreme discomfort in his hand. In early 2017, when I was performing the healing process for a woman in Mumbai the father of her, who was an 82-year old retired surgeon was watching me closely as I was working on. After she had completed her treatment I asked him if I could also help him.

He informed me that there was a lot of pain within his right hand. I looked around and was shocked to find that he didn't have a left hand. There was only a small little stub of his back arm, close to the shoulder. He explained to him that the left side of his hand needed to be removed following an incident in the past and that since then he has been suffering from intense pain in his hand. He informed me that this type of pain is common among amputees. It is known Phantom pain. It is a condition where his brain was still able to sense the the hand linked to his body and he felt high levels of discomfort. Even though he was taking a huge dose of painkillers each day the patient experienced a plenty of discomfort.

I accepted the offer to treat him, and as I imagined an arm that would be that was attached to his body I placed my palms in the air and began taking notes of the message from his hand as a result of sensations that my palm felt. After a while, I experienced a feeling with intense warmth and intense vibrations on my palms. I devoted all my concentration on the sensation.

This lasted for around five minutes and, during this, I kept asking him to see whether he could feel any signs of improving. At the end of five minutes, he said his pain had returned and was just as severe as it was it was before. It took me a few minutes more, and then decided to give up because there was no change. He was very sad, and returned in his room to rest. I was getting ready to go, but his daughter requested that I drink tea that she had made for me. I explained to her that I was disappointed that I was not in a position to assist her father.

Then her father came into the living room , and declared that his pain was been completely eliminated. I was stunned , and I asked him if his pain had diminished compared to earlier it, and he told me that there was no pain anymore. It was as if it was a miracle for the three of us who were sitting in the room. He looked extremely happy and content. I casually inquired about when he had been injured and he said it was in 2004. I was astonished to see the way a 13-year-old's pain went away in just 10 minutes of treatment.

Healing Experience 3: (Zero point Entrainment)

The healing process was carried out using an entrainment process that was based on an Zero Point state of a unfocused and still mind.

A student in my program of training suffered from neck and frozen shoulder and neck pain. He explained to me that his hands could not be raised beyond shoulder level, and was extremely painful if the hands were forced to go above. When he was on his seat, I sat behind him and entered the state of zero point conscious awareness (Explained within chapter 8). Then I gently pressed my fingers onto two of his shoulders. I connected the two points to three points of quiet in my body to induce the state of entrainment (Explained at the end of chapter 16) and remained in that position for a couple of minutes. Within about 4-5 minutes, I became aware and asked the man to examine his hands.

He got up from his seat then stretched his hands to the side, and then lifted his hands up. To everyone's and his own delight, both of his hands were straight and straight without any pain. He realized that in just five minutes, he successfully cured an issue that he'd had for a long period of. He explained to me that he tried a variety of therapies, medicines, and other treatments but had no effect I was astonished to learn that a five-minute treatment session led to him being completely free of the problem.

There are many other similar experiences I have discussed throughout this work. Some of them are covered in Chapters 14, 15 and 16, as well as the treatment method I used and the remainder are found in Chapter 20.

Then, I began regularly using the three methods on diverse issues, including digestive problems, Menstrual problems, Swellings Injury, Pain as well as ENT issues Headaches, Joint discomfort, skin problems emotional disorders, and even the early stage of Cancer.

The chapters that follow will present you with the principles of how healing methods work, as well as the step-by-step process to follow. I've tried to make it simple and simple so that you are able to test it for yourself or with others in a matter of minutes.

Chapter 4: Healing Principles

This chapter introduces the reader the Five Principles based on which Instant Healing works. I've figured them out after studying various healing methods and trying out the three methods described within this guide.

Although you can immediately heal someone without having these concepts (just following the instructions in chapters 14 15-16) I suggest reading these chapters to gain more understanding of these methods. You'll gain a lot of knowledge about the process of healing that will prove invaluable for the long-term.

I've tried to make this section simple and understandable by giving examples that are appropriate. It covers fundamentals and also the attitude and beliefs that are crucial for healers. It is important to note that the information given in this article may not be the 5% of what's actual happening. I've tried to record what I've personally discovered.

I have listed all 5 principles of healing below. A full description of each will be provided:

Principle of Healing 1. We all have Infinite Potential to manifest our wishes or heal someone else in the event that we create the perfect environment for it to occur.

2. Healing Principle: The healing when done at the most fundamental degree of our being i.e. the Zero Point, can create instantaneous changes on an emotional level.

The Healing Principle 3. Awareness can assist an individual body heal from any disease.

4. Healing Principle: When we are ailing, our body is trying to convey its condition to us. Listening to it will aid in getting the problem solved.

Healing Principle 5 Love is a powerful scalar energythat can bring healing on all levels.

The healing principles mentioned above basically work on the basis of a desire to heal. As far as the healer's perspective is concerned, he will certainly have an intention to cure. But, the person who is being treated must also have the intention of getting healed. The importance of intention is discussed in depth in Chapter 5.

***

In the next pages I've attempted to explain each fundamental principles of healing in detail.

Healing Principle 1:

We all have Infinite Potential to manifest our desires or heal someoneelse, as long as we create the proper conditions for it to happen.

On a fundamental level, we are composed of molecules and atoms and every atom is a bundle of an immense amount of energy within and if it is released (as in the case of an nuclear bomb) could cause the destruction of the entire world. At the very core of existence, all of us are powerful bundles. Every time, holy books saints, spiritual guides and saints have shared the same information. If this is true, why do we not see this in our lives? We aren't able to realize our dreams quickly.

In order to answer the question I'll offer an example. Take a look at this. When I throw a large rock or boulder in the very unstable Atlantic Ocean, do you believe it will cause ripples? It's absolutely no. This is due to the high turbulence in the ocean will not permit the stone's impact to create ripples. But, if I use an empty bucket with absolutely still water and drop small amounts of sand into it there will be ripples. Therefore, the capacity to cause ripples is not dependent on the size or the size of the stone, it is dependent on the quietness of the surrounding. If we can attain a STILL STATE of Being, then we will be able to manifest our dreams or help someone else or ourselves.

The state of being still can allow an intention to form waves, which results in the reality we wish for. Please take note of the term 'Still state Being', not "Still state of Mind". The Mind and the Being are two distinct things. Actually the Mind must disappear in order to be conscious that we are.

Thus, if we can gain an access point to quiet or no-mind even a tiny amount of intention is enough to cause ripples of change and could set the universe on the path to the goal you want to achieve.

Healing Principle 2:

Healing, when done at the most fundamental degree of our existence (The Zero Point), can result in instant transformation at the physical level.

It is essential to comprehend that the healing process being achieved through these methods is occurring on a higher level. So, let's first examine some of the most important points concerning this. Although our bodies appear consist of solid matter which is broken down into molecules and Atoms, quantum physics informs us that each atom is more than 99.99 percent empty space, and subatomic particles that move at lightning speed across the space are actually bundles of energy that vibrate. The vibrations they generate are not random or irrelevant. They carry information that determines how they move and the type of solid matter they produce. So, in essence our bodies are made of only information and energy.

Every Object that exists = Information + Energy

Every single thing in this universe is made by the exact same energetic energy however, at a different level of energy and certainly with a unique amount of data. It means that our body, stone or drops of water all possess the same basic energy building blocks in a certain amount. Based on the information code is associated with it the energy is able to take a particular form , be it the human body, stone, or even water.

Every cell in our body is made up of one single cell, which was created through fertilization. When the multiplication process began the cells were allotted the same amount of energy and information code, thus causing one cell into kidney cells that filter blood, while another cell will make an eye's retina eyes and another to create cells that make up the heart beating. Everything is controlled by a plan or pattern at the core that is the basis of all our lives.

This pattern aids in the transformation of the chaotic energy that are generated by the quantum field into meaningful , orderly pieces of reality. When the pattern can affect our body in a positive way and effectively, the balance of information and energy will be maintained, which will lead to healthy and well-being.

To function effectively, a mobile application requires connectivity to the internet and synchronized with databases on the server, and has to be maintained regularly. To be healthy, we should remain connected to the source of energy. Ensure that we stay in sync with the database pattern and receive regular updates throughout our lives.

If for some reason, we are not able to stay in sync in the pattern of the universe then the information and energy code becomes outdated or disrupted. That's when diseases occur. For instance cancer cells possess the same amount of energy as normal cells, but they have a different informational code that has been altered or distorted and causing problems.

Simply put healing someone involves aiding them in synchronizing their own being to the universal code of Energy + Information. This synchronization occurs when we are in the zero point of existence.

The Zero Point state refers to the state that is 99.99 100% emptiness, or Nothingness or Vacuum, in which quantum particles are all present. If we are able attain this state, it's possible to synchronize any individual with the energy source that is universal, for healing to occur instantaneously. I've discussed more of this later in chapter 8 that deals with the method that is known as zero Point Entrainment.

Let me explain how this condition can trigger instant healing. In accordance with the principles of problem-solving, to tackle any problem it is essential to be at least one step lower. This helps us tackle the root of the issue. When it comes to healing the body, this means that in order to fix any issue with our body, it is necessary to work on the deeper levels. And the more deep we go, the better is the healing. When we get deeper and deeper, healing will become ever more lasting comprehensive and holistic.

So, if we wish to treat a body, we must go to the Organ level. This is exactly where the surgeon is working through cutting, stitching or transplanting.

We could also decide to look at an individual cell level to resolve the problem. This is the place where Nutrition therapy, Naturopathy and Ayurveda would be effective.

If we decide to treat a deeper cell, we will need be treating at an Atom level. That's the place Allopathy, Conventional medicine or chemotherapy can be used.

If we want to go even into the depths, we'll need to lower our levels to a sub-atomic particles level (Nano-particle scale). This is how Homeopathy operates.

If we decide to go one level deep, we'll need to lower our levels to a Wave-level, because waves generate Nano particles when they meet. Therapies like Radiation Therapy, Color therapy, Light Therapy, Sound Therapy, Mantra therapy, etc. are based on the wave.

But, if we wish to get below the waves, and to the depths of existence, below waves, there is nothing.

It is a state where Emptiness is the Zero point.

The change that is created in the realm of nothingness is bound to have an effect that cascades over the waves. This will cause a change at the nano particle level the atom level, cell level or organ level and eventually the human body. All of the above occur instantly.

Since this process is activated on the fundamental level of building blocks, this creates an energizing change to the whole system i.e. the remainder of the body. So, this therapy does not trigger any adverse effects that could be present in other treatment at any other level that is higher than the zero point.

Healing Principle 3:

The awareness of one's body can assist it to recover from any disease.

An interesting, but not widely known fact about Awareness is that awareness or consciousness aids in healing and keeps the body into an equilibrium or equilibrium. When any body part is injured, sick or exhausted the body attempts to bring our attention to it.

To draw our attention to the area the body generates the sensation of pain at the location. This way, we instantly shift our focus to the area. The greater the awareness needed is greater, the more discomfort.

If, for instance, my knee isn't performing well in healing rapidly, it triggers pain in the knee which is why I concentrate my attention or focus there. If I focus on it with complete attention, my knee will heal itself quickly. I am confident in this statement after having performed hundreds of instant healings. Instead of being attentive to your knee, and offering the knee our complete attention then we tell it to stop by taking a painkiller.

This is the point where everything begins getting out of hand. The effect of taking a painkiller and removing the pain, is:

1. We're not conscious or even aware of our knee
2. We do not think we need to take it off. We continue to stress it with our usage, which damages it further.

I advise that people should look at the pain not as a cause, but rather as a way to solve the problem. If we experience any kind of sensation in our body, whether it pain, an itching or tingling sensation, if we simply pay attention to that area and let the body do what it needs to do in order to heal. When the problem is solved the discomfort that is a method to bring us into our awareness and bringing us closer to our bodies, will go away automatically.

Just paying attention to our body's needs regularly is a simple way to maintain a healthy lifestyle.

Healing Principle 4:

An injured body attempts to convey its issue to us. Listening to it could aid in getting the problem addressed.

Recent research has shown that in our bodies, when there's a defect within a cell, the cell communicates to other cells, and also to the brain, seeking the corrective action. Similar to this every time a person within this universe is suffering from problems, be it an issue with their health or other issue, their body will automatically communicate to the universe to resolve the issue. It could take forms of both verbal or non-verbal communications, which could be detected through our ears or sensed by other organs of sensory.

If someone is listening to this signal (on behalf of all the world) the issue instantly begins to be solved. Let's say a young woman is crying as she broken her favorite toy or doll. If we just provide her with a listener's ear and attempt to comprehend her issue or feelings, typically she will stop crying. The act of listening can be extremely therapeutic.

What else can counsellors do? They listen with great care and awareness. Issues typically are solved through their presence as an observer. Counsellors are not present to discuss issues or offer suggestions. They are not required to reply to your questions, make a decision, or give advice.

They are here to listen to and to receive information but not to distribute any kind of information. In contrast to other healing methods which healers are in a giving mindset and sending energy, in this method we don't send anything. Instead, we are in a state of receiving. We are receiving messages.

The only requirement is listening as closely and as intently as you can. We must remain focused, keep our thoughts, and our preconceptions awayand allow our attention to the person who is on behalf in the name of God. The healing will then happen spontaniously, just like the power of a miraculous event.

Healing Principle 5:

Love is a very potent energy that can cause healing on all levels.

Our heart produces a powerful Electro-Magnetic force, which is a scalar form of energy which can be used to heal. The scalar form of energy is an energy type that can be transmitted over any distance or in any direction without losing its power.

In his book "The Energetic Heart', McCraty clarifies that the heart produces the most powerful electromagnetic field within the body. The electrical field measured through the electrocardiogram (ECG) is around 60 times more powerful than brain waves that are detected in the electroencephalogram (EEG). Research has shown that this strong magnetic field could be observed and measured up to a distance of several feet from a body and also between two people who are within close proximity.

It is commonly referred to as LOVE. It isn't visible but it can be experienced as an emotional feeling. This feeling of Love , emanates from the heart Chakra and Anahat Chakra towards any part of our body that is ill, immediately initiates a healing reaction.

The love feeling, whenever it is directed in any direction, through our awareness and breathing can bring Energy and Order in harmony immediately. It is fascinating that this love energy can be transmitted to things like water, or even the metal of coins, and is then passed on to someone who requires healing.

I have extensively utilized the power of love to heal hundreds people who have been healed of numerous health issues in just 7 minutes of this potent positive energy projected onto them. Chapter 6 contains additional information on Love and Heart energy. The process of healing the Heart Energy is detailed in chapter 14.

***

The attitude and beliefs of a healer

In this article, I've described the mindset that one should develop to be a good healer.

The first thing we need to understand is that we are not the healers. The universe does the healing, and our part is limited to serving as an intermediary for healing to take place and nothing more. It is essential to not let our egos be a factor as it can happen quickly once we begin to experience results in healing. In the beginning, in January 2017, following the healing was successful an individual told me, "Hey Sachin, you appear to have special abilities" . Then a feeling of pride flooded my mind. But, I recognized that, if didn't manage this emotion, it could create an Ego and I had to keep this from happening at all cost.

It is important to remember that when our Ego is revealed the moment that we become isolated from our universe. Our connection to the universe, and also with the person we are healing disappears and healing ceases occurring. I've noticed that the less grounded I feel and the more in the state of gratitude and love for the universe, the better the healing process that occurs.

Therefore, I begin my session by clearly explaining to the person I am working with, that my purpose is to create the right environment where healing can occur. Because I'm not actively involved, I am not a part of any healing success as well as I don't need to be upset if healing does not occur. If successful healing results occur I thank God for helping me and thank God for choosing me to participate to the process of healing.

I inform people that their bodies will do the healing and my function is to be catalyst to assist the universe find them and to heal them. I stay in the state innocence and follow my intuition as that heal-related processes are concerned. If I trust my instincts and just follow the flow, I've noticed that it often leads to a positive healing result.

I began my journey into healing because of a desire to be of assistance to the universe and I have been helping those who seek my help with their health concerns. I strive to do my best to make them get better. I also strive to impart these techniques to everyone I can.

I'd like to conclude this chapter by reiterating love, caring, compassion acceptance, humility, Selfless Service and Surrender are the core values for those who want to become healer.

***

***

Chapter 5: A Plan To Be Healed

Intention is the beginning point , or the root of all that is created in the world. Stephen Covey has said that each creation takes place twice. The first time it happens, it is within the mind, as an idea or intention while the second one takes place in the real world. The intention of our mind determines where the creative energy is concentrated and how it manifests.

The intention is what is the first step in any decision. Let's suppose that I wish to drink water and thus want to lift the glass of water that is placed before me. In the milliseconds that pass before my muscles in my hand begin to move and the physical hand movements occur there is an intent that exists that makes everything happen automatically. Once the intention is present and the hand is moving, it happens naturally. I don't have to be conscious to get my hand moving there. Like that the universe is fueled by our intention.

A lot of you have observed that when we are pursuing the goal or objective, and we're passionate about it, often the path to reach the goal is laid out before us and we begin moving towards that direction.

There's a reason behind to the reason this is happening. In our brains, there is a system known"the Reticular activation system (Let's refer to it as RAS). This RAS is the one that connects us to what we're trying to locate. To illustrate of this, suppose I'm planning to purchase a certain vehicle within the next few months, such as an Silver Coloured Honda Civic, and I have set that goal, over the next few days, I begin to see Silver-coloured Honda Civics all around me - on roads in the Toll Plaza and in parking areas, in shopping complexes, and even in my neighborhood. These were all never seen previously.

The cars were clearly present, but I was not paying attention to them. When we activate the RAS gives our body what we should be aware of. The intention is the starting point. Without an intention to create, creating can not begin.

Additionally, the intention needs to be made known to the universe in a way that Universe can comprehend it. For example when I'm helping someone heal their knee pain and I believe that the knee will be healed soon, the universe can't comprehend this intention since it's expected to occur in the future. The universe can only comprehend the present moment and it doesn't know the future. Therefore, I need to set an end goal to ensure that the knee is 'healthy and the person is in good shape to walk'. This will be a success since it's written as a present-tense statement that is understood by the universe.

In the last chapter, under the subject of Healing Principle 1 I gave an example of dropping a rock in water , with the aim to cause ripples. The intention is similar to the stone. It should drop into the water that is still. There is no need to throw it forcefully. Dropping it on the ground is good enough. Keep in mind that during this process there is no effort required Everything happens and should occur easily. Flowers bloom effortlessly, while rivers flow easily. Everything that is based on universal principles can be done effortlessly and quickly. In healing it is also our desire to go from a state of 'Disease to one of 'ease'.

When we have set an intention to heal and set a healing intention, we don't need to think about how the healing will occur. It is not necessary to think about what should occur first and what will happen comes next. The universe is aware of what it needs to do and will work out the process. When an intention is in position, it will begin working with its infinite power to make that object that we desire in our lives.

Intention is the seed that started creation. The seed contains all the elements required to grow. It already contains each of the fine details, as well as intelligence or design necessary to allow the plant to develop into a tree, and then blossom. Just dropping an intention into the ocean of unlimited possibilities and endless possibilities is enough. Then , the cosmic intelligence determines how to organize the world to bring about peace prosperity, health, wealth and happiness immediately.

Do we have to believe in this to make it be effective?
I have a solution: ...'NO'

I've seen cases in which people didn't believe that it could work, but it worked for them.

The reason why these techniques are effective despite the negative beliefs within the mind is because it is a belief that exists in the realm of the Mind and these methods operate at the level which is more profound than the level at which the mind is. Actually, these methods are not related to the mind, and operate at a level that is deeper than that is where the universal spirit lives. They work regardless of whether one doesn't believe in these methods.

Let me provide you with an illustration. A person once was in the cafeteria at my clients office in Mumbai in which I had been conducting an session. He asked me to conduct an acupuncture session for his neck discomfort. When I asked him about the details I was told that he'd seen me just a month earlier and that I had conducted an hour-long therapy session with him. I was unable to recall the details the details, so he explained the details.

A month ago, while I was in his office to lead an event, his colleague was telling him about my ability to heal. Because he was skeptical in this claim and was a bit skeptical, he ridiculed it. The man was dealing with back pain, so to show the other person that such treatments do not work, he came to me after my lunch break and wanted to have an appointment to heal. Because I needed to begin my session right away and had no time, I offered him only 60 seconds of treatment.

A month later I received a request from him to come back for another session of healing because the 60-second treatment provided him with a substantial relief. Around 70-80 percent of his pain had disappeared. The time had come, he came to me fully aware of the fact that these healing methods work, and they can be effective even if one does not believe in these methods. I was delighted to provide him with a five minutes healing session. After that the patient was completely relieved from the issue.

***

Chapter 6: The Role Of Love In Healing

Love is a crucial part of the healing process. The sensation of love delivered to an injured body can immediately trigger healing. In this article, I will attempt to explain some of the most important aspects of Love.

The love I am talking about is not restricted to the typical love for the person we usually use to describe. It's not the kind of feeling of love when we feel physically attracted to someone else, nor the feeling we experience when we cry out in a show of compassion. It's something inherent and In the form of a sensatIon that Is shared by each and every living thing on this planet. The simple act of paying our the attention of a child who is playing, is interpreted by the child as a gesture of loving.

True love can only be felt by removing our minds and ego off the picture. The mind is a judge of separation and then becomes judgemental. When we put the mind off, then can we feel the profound love we have for ourselves and all that surrounds us. I was blessed to go through an awakening moment a couple of several years ago, when I was able to catch an insight into this profound sensation of pure unconditional love. It's something is very difficult for me to express in words. I will however tell you a little about it.

A little over 25 years ago one day I was working on some Spiritual practice of grounding following the instructions on a site. As I sat at my computer I was doing the steps given. I could see light emanating from the sun, passing into my chakra of the crown, moving through the remaining 6 chakras , before returning to the heart of earth. Then, I could see the energy manifest in the form of white light rising up and then descending towards me through the body before going back down in loops. From the heart chakra I imagined the bright and beautiful beam of white light that covered my entire body.

It lasted for around five minutes, and then and completely out of the blue I had a intense experience of awakening spiritually. It was an experience I will never forget in my entire life. It was an incredible sense of joy, but , at the same time there was a lot of paradoxes. I felt like I was not there, yet it appeared as if I was everywhere. I was less than the smaller, but nevertheless, I was larger than the largest. There was no starting place for me and there was also no final point. In the miles below, there was only me, and above, there was nothing but me. Everything else around me was me me alone.

The whole experience had resulted an experience of non-duality (Advaita), i.e. an experience of being one with all that was within me. Then, I experienced an intense sense of Love. It was something I'd never experienced before. It was an experience that was incredible, beautiful extraordinary, divine and unifying. It was pure love and unrestricted. It was everywhere and did not care on my surroundings.

I frequently experience this feeling of love whenever I am in an ethereal state which is a state that transcends the feeling of Separation from other people in the universe. It is more than an emotion. It is actually the very essence of who we are.

Love is the energy of Scalar energy that moves across all directions and travel over vast distances quickly. From what I've learned, scalar energy works over time and space. It creates a feeling of love that emanates from our bodies is the beginning point of this healing procedure. If this love is directed at the person in need with the intention of healing the body, it creates a deep relationship between the person who heals and the patient receiving healing. It also increases the healing process and provides immediate results.

I have noticed that this love feeling naturally occurs when healing healers enter the state of no-mind i.e. The zero point. If one doesn't feel this sense of Love in the natural way, it could be brought in artificially by contemplating a loved one that is dear in your life. It could be your children or your parents, close and beloved ones, or perhaps a kitten or puppy kitten that you feel a an overwhelming feeling of the love of your life.

It is beneficial for a healer to take the time to create this feeling of affection in the heart area before beginning with the process of healing.

I typically hold the person who is healing with my hands and, with my eyes in loving contact, I share my deepest feelings of love and affection for the person being healed. You can even give them a hug in the beginning of the healing process. This helps increase the feelings of love which speeds healing.

I believe that any person who has an unwavering affection for other people (be be it animals, humans or even plants) will be capable of healing quickly. Our love for our loved people is apparent. However, once we begin to feel the unconditional love and compassion towards strangers, the day will come when our hearts will begin to open and love will pour into every healing practice we can attempt.

Chapter 14 will guide you through the process of healing by using the energy of the heart, love. I have extensively utilized the energy of love for healing hundreds of people and experienced remarkable results in a short time. Try it out and you'll be surprised.

***

Chapter 7: The Process Of Awareness Is The First Step To Healing

Studies have shown that consciousness (or consciousness) is a state of consciousness that can cause a significant alteration in the way in which the universe works.

Have you heard about the double slit research? It is an intriguing element that is quantum mechanics. Here are some facts to refer to.

Quantum mechanics provides the finest theory we have to explain the world at the basic scale of atoms and subatomic particles. Perhaps the most well-known of its mysteries can be the idea that the result of a quantum test can alter, based on the decision made to measure or observe characteristics of the particles that are involved.

When the "observer phenomenon" was first observed by the quantum theory pioneers They were extremely concerned. It appeared to challenge the foundational assumption of every scientific discipline: that there exists an objective reality that exists beyond our perceptions. We know that how the world functions is contingent on the way we consider it as such as well as how we perceive it. Researchers were they were forced to conclude that objectiveity was a figment of their imagination, in addition to the fact that awareness i.e. awareness must be given to play an active part within quantum theories.

The scientist Pascual Jordan who collaborated with quantum expert Niels Bohr at Copenhagen around 1920 explained it this way: "observations not only disturb the measurement process but they also generate the results... It is our job to force quantum particles to assume a certain place." Also, Jordan said, "we ourselves generate the results of our measurements." All of this suggests that the universe acts differently when it is subjected to awareness, observation or awareness.

Awareness is the most important factor in healthy living. In all healing practices, one thing is universal and it is the presence of consciousness in the human body.

It is the term used to describe consciousness. When we are aware of something, it accomplishes two things. The first is that it immediately aids in the process of removing our mind , and also helps us to be conscious of our real nature the soul or spirit. More and more advanced levels of awareness can produce a very blissful experience that I've personally had. It's as good as the feeling one experiences when experiencing an intense gasp.

Joy or happiness is the real nature of our soul, and being aware is extremely beneficial when we're healing ourselves.

The second benefits of being conscious is when we are fully conscious, our mind goes still and we immediately begin in a state of stillness that is known as the Zero Point. When we reach the Zero point and we are in the perfect environment to allow healing to take place as I described earlier in this article.

Being aware greatly aids as awareness is the thing the body requires to heal. Once we realize this, the healing process will automatically and naturally begins without needing to take action.

Do you notice that when our bodies hurt using a balm can help and we get better after a short time. Have you ever considered the reason for this? The reason I see is quite simple. When we apply a balm we begin to feel a powerful cooling sensation and tingling wherever the balm is placed and, as a result, we are more aware of the area. The act of feeding it with awareness will help us feel healthier and recover quickly. Similar to when we apply a menthol-based lozenge to ease our throats or apply a Vaporub on our chest whenever we suffer from cold or cough. It helps us feel better.

One interesting thing to remember is that when your body requires awareness, regardless of whether you yourself create it accessible to your body or if'someone else' provides it to your body, it isn't a matter of importance. Your body will readily accept the awareness, and swiftly recover itself. This is because consciousness is not dual. It is one and is part of the universe. There is nothing that can be compared to 'Your awareness My awareness'. The observer could be different , but awareness remains the same in its uni-ness.

The consciousness that I carry is identical to the consciousness that runs through you. We ourselves are nothing more than a bundle of consciousness. Based on the frequency we vibrate at, the molecules and atoms of our bodies are moved and reorganized at the quantum level to shape our minds as well as our bodies. If we can alter the levels that we are conscious of, it is possible to create profound changes in our lives.

As healers We bring our awareness towards the physical body of the patient being healing in order that healing can begin. I've noticed that when I am at the zero level, even if take a look at a damaged body part, I immediately notice healing registers that are nothing but signals that indicate that healing is beginning. Awareness is definitely very effective in healing.

In Yoga exercises too the main concept is to perform every posture while being aware of every move. This is why it is advised to perform these yogasanas or poses slowly and with full concentration or attention to the. In reality, you'll be able to observe that if you complete any task at a slower pace it will be able to operate with greater awareness. This is the reason that in the many ancient practices, such as Tai Chi or Qi Gong that they practice slow-motion to increase awareness.

Do this now, and you'll be able to experience similar results to the ones above. Put your hands on the table with your palm facing down and affixed to the table. Then, move your hand up very slowly. It should go up millimetres by millimetres until it reaches the height of a foot over the table's surface. Then, in the same manner you can lower it to the table extremely slowly. When you are done you will notice that you've achieved a deep consciousness.

How do you know this? It's easy to discover. When you are at a high level of awareness, your brain is completely still. There wouldn't be any thoughts and your mind would not be bouncing around in the past or into the future. You'll feel a certain peace and tranquility within. You may even feel feeling of tingling in your palm due to the elevated awareness. Try the palm lifting and lowering exercises to see if you feel this.

When practicing Yoga Nidra, one is advised to relax and nourish the whole body with awareness , starting from the toes all the way to the head. Continually spending time with each body part feeding it in a mindful manner. Doing this will result an incredible relaxation, release from stress , and also healing.

***

Chapter 8: Zero Point Of Stillness

Zero is considered to be the most profound dimension of our existence which is where a single intention will manifest into reality which is why healing happens in a natural and effortless manner. But, in order to comprehend how to achieve zero point Zero point, first we must understand our mind as well as what it means to be in the state of 'no-mind' existence.

This chapter is split into two sections. In the first I've discussed the fascinating elements of our Mind and the way that it can cause turbulent conditions, which can impede our ability to manifest instantly. I also have explained how we can cause the mind to disappear at will in order to reach a 'No Mind state.

In the next part I will provide three steps to attain the Zero Point state of stillness and peace in only two minutes, moving to higher levels of consciousness. In this point that the magic of healing takes place.

Part I: Understanding our MIND

Let's attempt to discover the MIND. The mind functions as software inside the hardware we call our brain. The mind aids us think, think, think, analyze, and plan out our lives. It's like a useful tool in our lives. Like any other device or app is required to be turned on in order to use it and then has to be turned off once we are finished using it. Unfortunately we've neglected to do this in our minds.

In our youth when we needed to concentrate, we switched the Mind "ON" like an Radio set. However, in the years since, we've lost sight of that it must be shut off when it is not needed. Thus, the Mind, much as a Radio set, is constantly playing in the background moving from one program after the next. I'm sure you may have felt the mind that is running with thoughts and thoughts that never stop. It's hard to keep it quiet or unoccupied for a couple of seconds. It's like watching an animal jumping from branch to branch constantly. The most frustrating part is that we begin to associate us with Mind and its constant stream of thoughts, and then forget about the true self we are.

The Mind is a competent 'Servant' but an extremely poor 'Master'. When we are able to manage our mind the mind, everything is in order. Once the Mind begins to control us, the issue begins. For the majority of humanity, we have taken place wherein all of us have been conditioned to believe that 'We' are our Mind instead of our 'being We're unable to imagine our existence without the presence of the Mind.

The mind's constant flitting from one thought to the next causes so much turmoil in the sea of our existence that , no whatever size of stones of intent we drop into it there won't be any ripples made. Thus, shutting down the mind is the goal we must to accomplish, in order to achieve our dreams.

Remember that our mind is conditioned and infected with various assumptions and limitations. This limits our abilities, and eventually people begin to believe that they are normal people who are incapable of achieving miraculous things. By turning off our mind will help us discover our true potential.

Being able to move beyond our mind as well as aiding in healing , it can allow us to experience genuine happiness and joy that is our primary nature. To see our authentic self, we have to shut off our minds for a time.

This isn't an easy task because many people make the error of using their thoughts to shut down their mind. How do you get an instrument that is broken to repair it? How can the mind assist us go beyond the mind? It's not that simple. Therefore, moving beyond the mind or taking a step beyond the mental realm is to be done not using our mind and brain, but rather by making use of our body or consciousness.

In this article, I'd like to discuss a crucial aspect of the Mind that we have to comprehend. There are three distinct zones that we usually recognize as. The first is the Past and the third can be described as The Future and the thirdone, which only a small percentage of folks are familiar with is the "NOW",, or the "Present Moment". We're not usually conscious of it because when we are aware of it, it is like it's been relegated to the past. But, the present is where our whole life is. It's the truth. What is the Past as well as the Future are illusions that can only be comprehended by the Mind and not by the universe. The universe is able to only know one time zone which is "NOW".

The most interesting aspect is that the Mind does not exist currently. It simply disappears. The mind, aware that it doesn't exist in the present moment, constantly attempts to stay within it's Past or Future in the place where it can have some existence. So, throughout the day, our minds keep drawing us into the past and pondering about the events of the past or into the future and worrying about the possibility of something happening.

If we are able to connect to the moment in which we are, we can not be able to go back into the future or past and, once at the present the mind will be in silence and vanish.

There is a further benefit that we enjoy when the mind goes away. It is widely acknowledged that the mind is the cause of an abundance of emotional turmoil that can lead to various health problems. According to research, the majority of ailments that are physical in nature level are related to issues with the emotional part of. The majority of health issues are psychosomatic in origin (Psyche is the word for mind and Soma is the word for body). Many of the psychosomatic disorders will disappear when we understand how to control our mind.

The technique to make the Mind to be silent is quite simple. All we need Is to anchor it to the proper location. Let me offer an example. In order for a boat to stay steady at a specific place in the ocean we just need to anchor it to a point which will always be present at the exact area. If we also want our lives to be in the present (Present Moment) then we need be anchored to something that is within The Present Moment (NOW), every moment. But is there such thing?

The answer is easy. Our BODY is the only thing that exists solely in this present. Even though it existed before yesterday it was present in the present moment of yesterday. The same is true for our breath. at the NOW. The actions we do occur within the NOW. Do you believe that eating food can only happen at the moment. Similar to the process of walking and driving, gardening and cooking and so on. or more precisely, any activity is only possible in the present. This means that if we attach our attention to any of the above mentioned things or actions, then we immediately be immersed in the present moment.

Of all these, one of the most effective is to keep our attention towards our BODY as our body is always available anytime in contrast to cooking, driving or eating, in which we are both in motion and movement, it is much easier to stay aware of our body, especially when we sit still or seated.

So, 'Body Awareness is an easy method of bringing us back to the present. In the beginning, it might be difficult to keep your body in focus for more than 20-30 minutes at a time. The mind begins to take over and then starts to whirl around. In this situation we must keep reminding ourselves to be conscious of our body once more. However, over a long amount of time, one can be able to stay conscious of their body for longer periods of time, such as 2 or 3 minutes at one time. After this it is then that we are stuck in the present moment and the mind disappears, paving the way toward the Zero point. Moving a few levels further in consciousness then leads us directly towards the zero point.

I've already told you that to achieve an effective healing process you need to be in an State of Stillness and The Zero Point. It is evident that shutting off the mind can fulfill both of these conditions that can instantly trigger healing. An easy intention to heal someone will quickly result in changes in the physical body of the individual being healing. I've witnessed these changes taking place through joints moving around, gases being released, and joints aligning to their proper positions instantly.

Part II: Getting to The Zero Point state of Stillness and Bliss

This brief journey is comprised of three easy steps that are explained below. Note that after you've walked this route more than a few times, you'll acquire the capability of reaching the Zero point immediately and won't have to repeat these steps each time.

It is crucial to keep in mind in this regard is that the primary aspect that has to have throughout the entire process is awareness. Without this awareness our journey, we'll never be able to achieve anything.

Here's how you can accomplish it.

First Step: Awareness of Joy:

Be aware of your body for about 2 minutes or more. Being aware is simply paying your attention on your body parts individually or all together. The best way to do this is to sit in one spot and be aware of your body, breath as well as the clothes touching your body, the body touching the chair, etc. Just do this for about 2 minutes or longer and you'll feel a sense of joy in your body as well as your mind. It's typically an inner calmness and peace. you'll experience within only a few minutes.

It's often an overall feeling of happiness, when your thoughts are significantly decreased. There is a soft look on your face. In order to achieve this, simply keep an eye of your body or whatever slow movement you're doing. Simply rubbing your tongue toward the upper lip of your mouth is enough to bring us to awareness. Doing this will help to deeply connect our attention to Nowand the Present Moment, and create feelings of joy.

In essence, to take a look at step 1, sustaining BODY AWARENESS for a short period of time brings joy. In this point, we are prepared to move on to step 2.

Step 2 2. Peace to Stillness

Be aware of the feeling of joy you experienced in step 1. It should last for a couple of minutes or longer. Within a few minutes you'll feel a sense of calm and a profound feeling of peace within you. You will experience a feeling of being very still and centered. You will feel calm and serene. You may feel safe, secure and as solid as the rock and extremely stable.

It will feel like you are now immovable. This sensation is particularly felt in the lower region of the body, or near the base of the spine, where we feel more at peace. In conclusion, step 2: Maintaining awareness of JOY results in the feeling of STILLNESS. We are now prepared for step 3.

Step 3 Step 3: Stillness to the Zero Point

Simply be aware of the STILLNESS you are experiencing in the last the space of a period of time, around 2-3 minutes, you'll experience a peaceful state of no-mind. It is a state of mind where you may experience a complete lack of thought, an absence connection with the Ego as well as a sense of safety and oneness with everything else around. This is a sense like Unity (Advaita which is also called the state of non-duality) in the Universe.

It is usually an ethereal feeling, and you may feel like you're infinity. There is no beginning, there is no end, you are simply there and unified with all that is around you. There is a sensation of stillness, a feeling of being deeply connected to the energy of all things as well as a sense of being at one with all of us and a blissful sensation as a result of no-mind. It's a state of mind where we connect with our soul. To summarize step 3, maintaining the awareness of STILLNESS can create the ZERO point.

To summarize these three actions:

1. The awareness of the body leads us to Joy
2. The awareness of joy leads us to Stillness
3. Awareness of Stillness transports our to Zero Point.

When you have learned how to attain the Zero point, and have been successful at least a couple of times you'll notice that the process becomes simpler as your consciousness learns to recognize the triggers of each state with ease i.e. Awareness of Body stillness, joy and awareness. You'll learn how to spontaniously and effortlessly enter the Zero point in a short time and at a whim.

Finding the zero point is what meditation is about. But people make it that difficult that the majority of people are lost in the complexities of processes as well as rituals, singing, guided visualizations, etc. If you can get to the zero point frequently your life will transform into bliss. Anything that's not in order will be brought back in order.

If you do this consistently and over time, the peace and joy will be an integral aspect of your life and you'll be able to feel this throughout the day every moment. After this, those who are simply aware of your presence close to them physically or mentally will feel healing instantly. I've had the pleasure of hearing of a patient who was healed just by calling him.

In Chapter 16, you'll learn how to utilize the Zero point state to create an extremely effective healing method known as Entrainment.

Benefits of being at the Zero Point:

There is an immense advantage one can enjoy when they reach the zero point. When you are at this point, because there is a complete absence of the 'Mind' our body is completely free from any Psychosomatic diseases.

You may be aware that a large portion health issues stem because of our religious beliefs. In our daily lives we develop certain beliefs that can cause us to be afflicted because of health issues. For instance, if a person believes the consumption of Ice cream causes sore throat the next time someone consumes Ice cream and eats it, they will surely be suffering from sore throat. A lot of health problems like Allergies , etc. have their roots in our beliefs. When we reach the Zero point, due to the demise of the Mind the beliefs we hold no longer restrict us or influence us. A few minutes spent in the zero point each day is extremely beneficial for one's spiritual physical and mental health.

***

***

Chapter 9: Listening Can Be Therapeutic

Have you noticed that when there is a problem and we are feeling better when there's someone listening to us? In many cases even if another person is just listening but does not take action or offer a solution, just the act of listening gives us a sense of relief. Similar to when our body is sick or has a health issue and it needs us or someone else , to pay attention to it. It makes a statement hoping that someone else will pay interest to it. The message is targeted at the person suffering from the health issue and also to all the world.

I was recently exposed to an interesting idea known as 'Holding the Space'. It came from an article by Maryam Hasnaa. She wrote that "A Healer is not able to cure you. A healer provides space for you as you awaken your inner Healer in order to recover yourself"

The healer is the one who holds the space and healers simply create an atmosphere of silence, tolerance, and openness in which the pure listening that is non-judgmental takes place. It's a place where those who are keen to speak has the freedom to express without interruption, judgment or rebuttal. This allows every part of the message to be fully absorbed by the unconditional vacuum provided.

This is the space healers must create and be able to hold for the person that requires healing. When the healer has held the space that is created, the mind, body and soul that are ready to express itself, naturally makes use of this space for expression and heal immediately occurs. Who holds the space and listens to the message is irrelevant. If the individual himself or herself listens, it will aid in healing. Even if someone else is listening to the signals, it'll still aid in healing. The universe works in a non-dual fashion Therefore, 'Your awareness My awareness' and 'Your awareness' are the identical. Healing will take place regardless of who is listening.

The "listening" that I'm talking about is a state of receptivity that we experience as our own being or. When we listen to an audio signal the eardrums of our ears are receiving sounds of a certain frequency i.e. the frequency of sound waves. In order to "listen" to heal and healer, we place this type of receptiveness to our palms to receive the message or signal. It is during that state of openness the signal or message released by the body in pain is able to be detected by the healer, thereby triggering the healing process immediately.

The only thing we need to remember is that our body is sending us messages using an unrelated language to the human language we typically listen to. It's a language which must be felt or felt with the sensory organs of our body. When I am healing someoneelse, I usually sense this message, using my palms' skin that I am capable of feeling by way of various sensations like vibrations sensations of heat, tingling, etc.

Let me share an intriguing insight that I gained about this communication that provided me with a profound understanding of this communication. I was healing someone's back by sensing the body's signals through vibrating my palms. The other person, who was close by, unexpectedly fell into a state of trance for a short period. It was likely because of the healing environment that was created there. He was then being able to observe the healing process take place on a different plane of consciousness. He began talking about the way he could perceive the various organs in his body, and also how he was able to observe the healing process taking place.

After a short time after which he woke up from the trance, he told me that he saw an unending stream of information that he could see running from the back of the patient to my palms, then from my palms towards my body. When I inquired about what it was like, he told me it was like the light of a white beam and that the language used was not the way we recognize, but something completely different that was being encoded and decoded by the bodies of both individuals i.e. myself, who was the healing practitioner, and the person receiving healing. This is when I realized there was some sort of communication which was occurring in both ways. The more I could listen to it, the faster the healing process.

If I am saying that listening can be therapeutic and can lead to healing there are three ways in which healers can listen to someone who is in need of healing.

Hearing Method One: Paying attention to the words spoken by the person i.e. the words spoken that is later understood by our brain.

Listening Method 2. Listening to the body language of an individual by looking at them.

Listening Method 3. Listening to the communications of the individual's Bio Field that is felt by our fingers.

Listening Method 1. This is the method that we typically employ when someone is struggling that is physical or financial. We listen to them until they are able to feel more relaxed. A counselor, coach or guide would therefore listen to and assist the individual comprehend the issue or find solutions, accept the facts or take an take action.

Listening using Method 2 is when we watch how a person's body speaks to an individual, i.e. gesture, posture eye contact or body movement, through our eyes, and attempt to comprehend the individual.

But, in contrast to the two above I have discovered that listening method 3 aids to heal in a superior way , as it lets the healer 'Hold the Space to heal in the most effective way. Let me explain. Method 1 and 2, as we listen to spoken words either spoken or in body, the mind is always in action, trying to analyze, perceive, interpret, or clarify things. In a conscious or unconscious way, we are drawn into the habit of providing instructions or explanations, justifications, and argument. The silence required for the 'SPACE' to be efficient for healing is not found in the pure form' needed.

However, when we practice listening methods 3 Listening Method 3, the biofield of the person is communicating with a language our brain and our minds can't comprehend. So, naturally the mind remains silent and the mind is able to open to a

Pure, Clear silent, quiet space which is vital to heal.

Three healing methods are described in chapters 14-15 as well as 16 in this publication The Healing Technique described in chapter 15 uses the method described above, of listening to the person's body by using our palms. The Healer , by virtue of being in a state of awareness, silence and in a state of listening creates the space where transformations occur instantly in the quantum level of existence.

In the past three or four years I've used these methods of healing I've realized that if I concentrate my sensory organs on the body of the person, or to the part I am working on it is immediately a shift or change I notice, and it is as if another person's body is communicating with me on an entirely different level. I make use of my eyes, my skin, ears , and intuitive sense to discern any signals that another's body is sending.

My eyes remain open during recuperating to make use of my entire vision (Focal and peripheral) to listen. My focus is on the area of the body that is healing and my peripheral vision is trying to detect body micro-movements that are often observed in your body or the person who is being healing. The movements usually take their form of the twitching fingers, movements of hands or legs, or changes on the face , or the speed of breathing. In this way, I can pay attention to my partner's body language with my eyes.

I also pay attention to communications from the body of another by using my skin. i.e. I am keenly trying to discern all signals (in forms of tiny sensations) that the palms of my hands and my arms, or any other body parts is picking up. When I move my hands around the biofield of the person whom is healing me, I begin getting signals of communication the form of a tingly or scratchy feeling to my palms. a sensation of cold or heat or vibrations, a slight touch or tingling sensation, or tingling sensation, etc. This is the basic method of listening to the skin.

When I am in your healing, my sixth sense begins to receive signals that are that are a sense of intuition. Sometimes, thoughts come up in my head that are related to the disease or to a topic that provides me with a clue of what another's body's body's trying to convey. When I was in the process of healing an individual and each time I placed my hands on the throat chakra of her, she experienced an uneasy feeling and, in my gut, I sensed that she was repressing an emotion that she could not convey. The tears began to pour down her eyes. As I gently probed she began crying. She disclosed that she was involved in an affair prior to her marriage that she hadn't disclosed the man she was married to. When the process of listening took place she felt more relaxed immediately. This is an illustration of me paying attention to my sixth sense, or intuition.

While I provide the healing of clients, I feel that the body is trying to convey some message to God. As a healer, provide myself as a medium or channel for this message to reach the universe.

***

Chapter 10: Vata, Pitta & Kapha

When I first began my healing about four years ago, while I was aware of those three doshas (Vata, Pitta and Kapha) as they are defined in Ayurveda but I was not aware of the specific ways these are corrected and controlled throughout the healing process.

Different experiences in treating more than 600 people in the past four years gave me some interesting perspectives about this issue. Further reading has provided me with more ideas that I've discussed within this section.

Every cell of your body operates under three different regulatory systems, referred to as the Doshas within the Ayurveda system of medicine. The three Doshas are Vata Dosha, Pitta Dosha and Kapha Dosha. They are the Vata Dosha controls all kinds of movement within the body, Pitta Dosha controls metabolism and Kapha Dosha is responsible for the structure of the body. In the following pages, you'll be able to learn more about the different aspects that the above doshas represent. But the Vata dosha is described more in depth than Pitta as well as Kapha Dosha and are explained in a simple manner. There's a rationale behind the reason I've done this.

When doing healing for other people, receiving review of the healing process is crucial for healing practitioners. I've noticed that once changes begin to occur within our bodies, the first noticeable indications are those of Vata correction. These signals are easily felt in your body by the patient being healing, and may be seen clearly in the healing practitioner. The changes that result from Kapha Dosha or Pitta Dosha correction cannot be noticed or felt immediately as they take effect over a period of time. Because Vata correction provides us with an immediate feedback, knowing it is beneficial for the healer. This is why I've attempted to explain this in greater in detail.

To be healthy and live long the body requires Vata or movement that lets us breathe and circulate blood, transport water and food through our digestive system, urinary, and excretory systems in addition to sending nerve signals from our brain to all parts of the body. The body also requires Pitta, or metabolism, to take in air, food or water. Pitta is the digestive system that transforms complex matter into simpler matter, and aids in the production of the nutrients which are needed from the human body. In the same way, the body requires Kapha or structure to help hold cells together, and to form bones, muscle, fat ligaments, fibre, and bone.

Vata's seat of choice is in the colon i.e. the large intestine. However, it is also found inside the pelvic area the lower back and sacrum joints, thighs and the skin. Pitta's Seat is the Small stomach and intestines, while Kapha's Seat can be found in the chest. The three doshas are all necessary to construct the body and must be in good health to maintain the health of your. Here's a short description of the three Doshas symbolize.

Vata Dosha controls the movement of all the body parts from our toes to our heads. This includes the flow of blood and stools, urine as well as menstrual fluids, digestive fluids tears, saliva sweat, mucous as well as the osmosis that occurs between cells, and the movement of electrical impulses that travel through our nervous system. The flow is driven by a pressure that builds up that then pulls and pushes things around. If Vata is blocked or disturbed and the pressure build-up causes pain in various parts of the body. It can cause back pain, discomfort in muscles and joints as well as migraine, knee pain and more.

There are 10 different types of flow-regulating Vata or Vayu and could be classified into five primary types, and five subtypes. To make it easier, they are referred to in the following order: Pran, Apana, Saman, Udana, Vyan, Naga, Kurma, Krukala, Devdutt, and Dhananjay. Each of them is described below, along with some additional specifics.

1. Pran Vayu. Pran Vayu. Pran Vata or Pran Vayu is located in the heart or chest and controls the flow of breath into and out. It is the force that brings the senses to us. Its main site of operation is the brain. It is connected to the sense organs and the brain. The circulation areas in Pran Vayu

are the chest throat, throat, ear and tongue. It regulates the swallowing of food and sneezing. It also regulates Salivation, Sne and burping. It regulates consumption, inspiration, propulsion and forward motion.

2. Apana Vayu. The Apana Vayu is responsible for the downward movement, specifically the elimination of toxins and the faeces. Apana Vayu is also responsible for women's menstrual period. The lower abdominal region is where it's located which is the primary source of downward flow of the intestines as well as the reproductive tract and urinary tract. Cellular activity generates both the waste and work. Although Udana Vayu is in charge of doing the job, Apana Vayu is responsible to clean up the garbage. Apana Vayu eliminates waste primarily through the process of defecation and urination and menstrual cycle. Being the main source of downward flow of energy in the body, it's also responsible for the energy required to carry the baby from the birthplace out into the world.

3. Saman Vayu. This is the force of absorption. It is activated in the Nabhi Chakra or Solar plexus. Samana Vayu transports nutrients from the

intestines to the circulatory system. Likewise, the sensations that we touch are transmitted through the skin into Central Nervous System. If Samana Vayu is working well, all impressions are taken in. If it's in the state of dysfunction the absorption process becomes more difficult and malnutrition or numbness can be experienced.

4. Udana Vayu. It is located in the chest and is connected to the development of speech, growth & Expression Ascension, Upward Movement and Ascension. It is located in the regions that are located between the Heart and lungs. It is responsible for ensuring proper oxygenation of our body through breathing and maintaining both mental and physical alertness. Udana Vayu is also linked to information retention as well as alertness, memory and so on. In the direction of upwards, it operates in the regions which include the Nose, Navel, Throat and Neck and in the downward direction, around the diaphragm, umbilicus and diaphragm. It is involved in the expression of words, speech and singing. Udana Vayu is the one responsible for expression and action, which is that the energy received is put to work. Cells use the energy and carry out their

own duties. Nutritional elements are used to provide cellular energy as well as for the production of proteins. The nerves guide organs and muscles to function in a way that is appropriate.

5. Vyan Vayu. This controls the force that drives the reaction, shifting it from the center to the outer edges. The digestive tract is where blood transports essential nutrients through the whole body to ensure that each cell receives the adequate supply. Within the nerve system a signal transmitted from the central nervous system to a muscle or organ. Circulation of oxygen and blood in the body, sweat, the Reproductive fluids, seminal and sperm fluids, as well as water to different tissues and cells in the body. Vyan Vayu can also trigger movement in joints and muscles of the skeletal region. The contraction and relaxation of muscles are also controlled through this. It assists in bringing the sexual genital tract into the semen, and allows fertilization, implantation and conception.

6. Naga Vayu Naga Vayu is an Sub-Vata that regulates the flow in the mouth and throat. It also plays a role in Hiccoughs and burps.

7. Kurma Vayu: It's a Sub-Vata, which regulates the movement of eyes. The upward and downward and eye movements that are sideways and focusing, etc. along with the discharge of tears are as well controlled by Kurma Vayu.

8. Krukala Vayu The Krukala Vayu a Sub-Vata, which is located situated in the chest region. It regulates thirst and hunger. It also plays a role in the making a sneeze.

9. Devdutt Vayu It is a Sub-Vata, and it is a vata that operates from the nose towards the throat. It triggers a feeling of tiredness and triggers the process of crying.

10. Dhananjay Vayu The Sub-Vata is the most important one and is found throughout the body. It basically holds and pulls all cells of the body and body parts together. It is released from the body following death and results in swelling of the body following the death.

Pitta Dosha governs the transformative functions of the body i.e. digestion, metabolism or the breakdown of the body's elements in one form into another. metabolism, digestion or breakdown of things in the body from one form to another. Pitta Dosha balances the two elements that appear to be in conflict of water and fire. Together, they constitute the force of energy that regulates the body's transformative functions. its digestion, metabolism, and even hormones of the body are thought to be controlled through pitta.

Kapha Dosha is the governing force for the structure and lubrication of the body and mind. It regulates weight, growth and immune system, as well as the joints' lubrication and lungs, and the development of the seven tissues -- nutritive fluids fat, blood, muscles bones, marrow, and reproductive organs.

Of the three Doshas mentioned above which we mentioned in the past, observing Vata Dosha changes is easiest. When Vata dosha begins to become controlled and balanced, changes can be observed through different body movements that can be felt or observed by the patient as well as by the practitioner. I refer to these the Healing indicators. These healing indicators assist the healer receive immediate information during the healing session , and ensure that they are on the right path.

Feedback from Vata indicators can be very beneficial for our healing sessions as it helps us understand which areas to concentrate on and whether we're going in the proper way or in the wrong direction. Most of the time in the healing process it is when Vata pressure begins to move out of the body it begins moving from one part of the body to the next, until when it's out of the body by way of burps. One common thing I've noticed is that when a foot of a patient is painful, then after a time, when Vata begins moving the pain will shift to the thigh or hip, and disappears when the vata pressure releases through burps.

If I treat patients who have lower back pain the pain tends to shift upwards toward the shoulders or upper back until it goes away after a few burps. Neck pain is usually shifted toward to the area of your head. As healers one must recognize that pain shifting is a sign that healing process has begun, and it is important to pay attention to the new location in which pain has changed and keep doing it until the vata pressure decreases through burps.

A lot of people have told me that they feel a tingling and movement or flow within their bodies after I begin the healing process. Later, when Vata begins to regulate it is a sensation of gas buildup in the abdomen. I've noticed that at times gas isn't quickly released. In such situations, I must concentrate my attention on their abdominal region or the solar plexus area to allow the gas to release. If burps begin to occur, typically, I am confident that vata release is now in full swing. Vata releases either in a flash or within the next few hours.

Below are the signs of healing that I've encountered over the past four years. Certain of them can be noticed by the healer while others are perceived by the person receiving healing however they may not be visible to the healer.

1. The twitching of hands and legs
2. Fingers moving (Very normal)
3. The sensation of tinnying in your hands or on the legs

4. Burps (Very frequent for those who suffer from Pain)
5. Feeling of circular movements in abdomen
6. Feeling of something being pulled into your being.
7. Apathy in the hands or feet
8. Feelings of bubbles moving through the body
9. Eyeball movement
10. Salivation and the swallowing reflex
11. Eyes drooping
12. Eyes with tears
13. Change in the breathing pattern
14. Hiccoughs
15. Feeling of lightness, weightlessness
16. The sensation of cold or heat throughout the body
17. Pain shifts from one area to the next
18. A slight increase in discomfort
19. Eye blinks or a flutter of eyebrows
20. Twisting of facial muscles

If I see any of these signs, I am confident that Vata correction has begun, and that I am moving in the correct direction. So, during the healing process, I monitor these indicators. This is not just helping me keep my mind on track which is crucial during healing as well as guiding me on whether to continue following the same path or alter my method.

Often, I experience some sensations or signals in my body that could indicate that the healing process is creating an impact on the person who is being healed. There are times that when I'm healing people suffering from back or shoulder pain feel the sensation of burps throughout my body and the person I'm healing begins to burp as well, signalling that there is a Vata flow has been activated within his or her body. Once this occurs the pain will begin to decrease and usually disappears.

I've realized over the years that Vata trapped and accumulating within the lower back, or shoulder creates pressure, which can cause discomfort. When this Vata is released through burps, pain is gone. I've treated hundreds of people suffering from different types of pain in by this method.

When I first began to practice this healing method certain people complained that there were some side effects from this method of healing i.e. an increase in pain, shift of the pain to another part of the body or release of gas. All of these signals indicated the healing process was taking place and that the body was in the process of cleaning itself up. your body tried to shift Vata(gas tension) from one area to another until it was completely released from the body. In many cases, I found that after experiencing these effects for a short time it was not a further problem, and the result was complete relief from the difficulties which were initially encountered.

Healing power from the all-powerful, infinitely aware universe makes no mistakes. Sometimes, what we perceive as a problem in our limited vision can actually be a 'Healing Process Indicator' that results in solutions for the universe over the long-term. Remember that these aren't harmful consequences.

If you follow the methods of healing that I have described in the book, it is not just do the issue and symptom go away, but also the temporary manifestations of the healing process will also disappear within a short time.

***

***

Chapter 11: Health And Emotions

This chapter is about the emotional aspects of health and well-being. This subject is so vital that it should be the starting point to all discussions on health and diseases. Many diseases are by a unsettling emotion in our brains and the answer to these health problems is only possible when we consider this aspect. There are a lot of books, books of research and huge literature available on this subject.

The term Disease i.e. Disease itself provides an indication of what is causing the problem. If a person isn't at comfortable with something, it's likely to trigger a feeling of dis-ease. Being uncomfortable with anything, whether it's an event, a person or object, or something else can cause an unwelcome feeling or mental image within the mind.

If these thoughts or emotions are too intense, and we feel uncomfortable with things for a prolonged period and then it can lead to condition that is an illness that affects the physical body. The function that a healer plays is discover what the person does not like and then deal with the issue. If a person isn't at ease with a specific situation, there might be two approaches to deal with the issue. Alter the situation or at a minimum, ease the person's mind about the situation through changing their perception or belief. This is exactly what a counselor or a psychiatrist is likely to do.

I've realized in the course of three years in my therapeutic work that the root of the majority of diseases (especially those that modern medicine is not able to effectively treat) is due to emotional issues. Even those diseases which modern medical science claims to cure frequently return to patients in the same way or in a different form, as an indication of recovery. It is likely that this is because modern medicine is only concerned with symptoms, not the primary cause which, in many instances, is at a more emotional level.

We frequently try different kinds of treatments but with no result, but we aren't aware that the root of the problem lies deep within us and is manifested in the form of or other emotion, such as guilt, fear shame, sadness, anxieties, traumas and resentment, etc.

In the past two years, I've been treating a number of cancer patients. One thing I observed was that every patient had one or more or another emotional issue deep within their heads. In some instances I had to put in a much effort to assist people speak out about their feelings. As I conducted the healing session, I also realized the extent to which both the emotional and physical illness were interconnected.

In the last couple of years, I've been helping three women who were being treated for cancer. In the sessions of healing I was able to sense that the illness was connected to an unresolved emotional issue. When I spoke with them, they spoke to my about how they felt. In one instance it was an emotion associated with her son, in another it was an extra marital relationship and the guilt that comes with it. In another case it was anger that had led to tumors developing in her liver.

I once treated an individual suffering from extreme lower back pain and was experiencing a lot of discomfort in her abdomen. If I asked her, she stated that she felt it was like a knot, which was in her abdomen for a long time. It was a fascinating experience for me to learn from and I learned a lot about the role that emotions play in the development of the disease.

When I began treating her by paying attention to her body's messages using the palms of my hands, she was in a wave motion. Her abdominal region and chest began going between them. It appeared like she was experiencing convulsions. But when I asked her if she was experiencing some discomfort or not, she said that she felt at ease and relaxed. After a few minutes, tears began falling down her face and she began to tell me stories about her family, life, and friends. This included an extra marital bond which she has with a particular person, and the guilt she lives with in relation to this marriage.

When she continued to tell me this story the tears started rolling across her cheeks. However, she seemed to be getting improved and better. In just a few minutes she was smiling on her face. When I inquired about how she felt she said she felt that the backache was been completely eliminated and that the knot-like feeling in her stomach also disappeared. I was able to see that the clearing of emotional energy was the key to healing. I spoke with her a couple of weeks later, and she informed me that she had been completely healed. She was shocked at the way she had jokingly shared with me everything that she never had discussed with anyone else in her life.

Dongui Bogam Dongui Bogam is a Korean book written by the physician of the royal family, Heo Jun (1539 1639-1615) and first released in 1613, during the Joseon Dynasty of Korea. The Dongui Bogam contains the following information: "Liver is in charge of anger, the heart is responsible for happiness, spleen the one responsible for thought the lungs take care of sadness, while kidneys are responsible for fear."

The book "You can Restore your Life written by Louise Hay is one of the most insightful books I've come across in the field of how emotions affect our health. It offers a comprehensive list of health issues and how they relate to emotions and feelings like anger, fear Resentment, Guilt, anxiety, and insecurity. and also offers suggestions on how to beat health issues by identifying the root causes of emotional issues and addressing these emotions effectively.

Healing takes place quickly at the Zero point because at Zero you are completely connected to the present moment and there aren't any negative emotions.

***

***

Chapter 12: The Overview Of 3 Methods

The book I've presented three methods for healing. Two of them are easy to master and you will see they are effective for anyone from day one. The third method will require the healer to attain the Zero point in silence and stillness before they is able to use this method. Although reaching this Zero point is simple however, one must do it several times before they are successful in healing oneself.

The three healing methods are listed below:

1. Healing with the energy of the heart of unconditional love
2. The body's communication is the key to healing. body's signals
3. The healing process is facilitated by entrainment at Zero point

Personally, I started using the healing technique 1, i.e. using heart energy to treat various ailments. To this day I have found it to be one of the best and effective technique to treat all kinds of health issues. Then I provided healing to lots of people by using the method of listening to body's messages. Today, having been in a position to attain the state of zero points quickly, I am using the zero point entrainment technique also.

Of the three methods, I choose to use healing through listening to the body's biofield typically with clients because of two reasons. One reason is that it is able to be done by not touching any part of the body receiving healing. The second reason is that, in contrast to heart healing,, it is simpler since heart energy healing requires deep breathing. This, if prolonged for longer periods of time may result in a little hyperventilation. This can cause some fatigue and dizziness when done for a longer time.

This is not the case when we heal through listening to our body's biofield. Additionally, the process is simple and does not make us exhausted. Entrainment at Zero point is most straightforward, but it is only possible when the healer has reached the state of being still and no-mind.

I would suggest that beginners should begin with Method 1 or Technique 2. When you begin to see results with these two techniques then you should attempt Technique 3. At this point, due to the application of techniques one and two, you could have experienced greater levels of consciousness and you'll be able to grasp the Zero Point state.

The chart below provides an analysis of the three healing techniques I have discussed within this publication.

Healing method 1 Healing method 2 Healing method 3
Description Healing with Heart Energy Healing by Listening to body's Healing Communication at the most profound levels of Zero Point
The method employed to create Healing Deep unconditional love when it is delivered to the body, causes healing. If a body is treated with pure awareness this creates healing. The process of bringing a body back to the state of

stillness through an entrainment process results in healing.

Important Factors: Feeling of Love and Oneness, as well as the caring and empathy of the healer for the person who is being treated. Intense and deep attentive listening from the healer, without judgement. The healer's state is of no-mind and Stillness , where thoughts aren't there.

Healing method: Breathing deeply and sending love through the Heart Chakra as a beam of bright light towards the body that is healing. The bio field of the body through its sensitivity. palms located close to the body that is being healed. Triangulation for entrainment to Zero Point, Triangulation with three points, with two palms touching the body, and the third zero point within the healer.

This type of treatment can be administered with no contact to the human body. This treatment can be used to provide distant healing by using a photograph or Icon. It can be done by not touching your body. This technique can be used to facilitate distant healing with a picture or an imagination. The need for physical contact is with two places on the body that are being healing. This can be used for remote healing with a photo.

Potentially cause mild hyperventilation as a result of breathing deeply for longer periods NIL However, Healer has to have reached zero Point in Stillness or else it will not work.

Making Healing Water through Quantum Charging Quantum Charging can create healing water. Charge water that can be used to aid in Healing not applicable to Zero Point water can be utilized to aid in Healing.

Remarks for Beginners: Technique for Advanced Beginners

Chapter 13: Guidelines Prior To When We Begin

Before we move on to the following three chapters, i.e. chapters 14, 15 16 and 17, which offer information on three healing methods It is crucial to know the aspects must be considered that can help aid in making the healing process more efficient.

This chapter's guidelines relate to the four following areas:
1. The choice of the best "Place" and "Time" during the therapy session.
2. Knowing the health issue that requires attention.
3. Conducting a brief 'Pre-Assessment' of the severity of the issue.
4. Understanding what to expect in the course of this healing process.
5. Do's and Don'ts' prior to and during the lesson.

Selecting the best location and timing:

For all three techniques of healing The choice of location is not an issue. The techniques can be utilized virtually anywhere indoors or out either standing or sitting, and even while traveling. Only requirement for both practitioner and the person who is being treated are able to position themselves in a comfortable position which allows the healer apply the technique successfully.

In the case of Technique 1, i.e. heart energies, the practitioner must send unconditional love from the heart to the person being treated. Thus, both can be located 10-15 or 20 feet from one another since the healer is only required to be able to see his or her body and the patient being treated. To be honest, being able to see the other person isn't necessary. I've successfully used it on people who were sitting in the same room. I also utilized remote healing.

If you are using Technique 2, i.e. healing through listening to the body's signals it is important to be close to of the healer because the healer must utilize palms to detect the body language of the other body. The person who is being treated may be standing, sitting or lying down. The healer may be standing or sitting close to them. So, staying in a distance of 3 feet is a good idea.

However, for using Technique 3, i.e. Zero Point Intrainment, the person who heals will need to be physically in contact with the person receiving healing and so a suitable posture to sit, stand or lying down needs to be selected. The healer could sit or stand at a comfortable level.

I have tried all of the above treatments at home, outdoors at offices, trains busses, trains airports, and almost everywhere else and have seen results that are positive. For technique 2, however I stay clear of areas where there are people watching , especially because the healing process appears to be an
A little odd with the healer's hands moving up and down in a manner that could seem odd to the other. I also inquire about the level of

comfort for the person receiving treatment. Some people aren't willing treatment in the presence of the public, while others do not mind.

Before beginning ensure that the location in which you're doing healing is safe for you as for the person receiving healing. If you can, ensure that there aren't interruptions from other people or the sound of the radio or television placed close by. The space where you will be performing the healing process should be comfortable, in terms of the atmosphere. It shouldn't be too cold nor too warm.

If you're using Healing Technique 2 i.e. healing through being aware of the bio field of the person using your hands, make sure that there's no blast of air coming from air conditioning units or fans that are directly coming into your body. This could hinder your ability to discern the message of the body of the person through your palms. Sometimes, the feeling on our palms are so subtle that it is difficult to recognize the signals when a large blow of air comes into our palms.

In terms of the exact time that healing should be completed I've never found any particular time in which healing shouldn't be carried out. Any time that is suitable for the healer as well as the person who is being treated. It is only necessary to determine whether they are in a good place and are not in a rush to get to another. In general, I make sure they have at least 15-20 minutes available. It is usually enough for the first session, but in some cases, one may want to do longer depending on how the body reacting. It could be necessary to devote more time should you decide to try a different method as well if the first method does not show the healing signs you want to see.

I suggest that you not schedule the healing session right after the person receiving healing had eaten lunch, breakfast, or dinner.
This is mostly because of the following motives
1. In the process of healing typically, it is when a Vata Dosha balance is achieved and gas begins to release from the body part affected and one

may have burps. It is difficult to let go of this gas efficiently if the stomach of the patient is overflowing.

2. Following a meal it is evident that the energy of the body is also transferred into the digestive system because digestion is an energy-consuming activity. Because of this, the person who is healing may be a little tired and the energy needed might not be available to the other parts of the body to allow to heal.

3. After eating large meals individuals typically feel drowsy and be less aware. Because these healing techniques are built upon awareness, it might be best to avoid this particular time. I've noticed that, as healer, too I'm not at ease when I perform an healing session right after an eating heavy meal.

In general I offer healing to patients prior to eating or after one hour of eating their meal. In the event that someone experiences an ongoing release of gas throughout the session, I advise them to consume a light, non-spicy meal for the next 8 to 10 hours. They should also consume plenty of fluids until the gas release has stopped.

The person who is undergoing the healing procedure should have had enough water and is not dehydrated. A well-hydrated body aids in regulating the flow of blood in the body, resulting in quicker healing.

Ideally, following a healing session, the patient should not experience a strenuous and stressful day, but let the body have some rest to recuperate. In this way I believe it is beneficial to conduct one session of healing at night, to ensure that the body of the patient can some rest before bed.

The health problem to be understood

Information regarding the health issue is essential since it assists us to gain an grasp of the problem, and also to ensure that we are able to establish an purpose i.e. the intention to heal in our minds.

I usually try to ask a few, or all of the questions below:

1. What health problem do you're facing? (A general description)
2. When did it begin and how long have you had this. (Is it a chronic or Acute disease?)
3. What are the symptoms You have seen (Past and present)
4. Have you received any kind of treatment?
5. If so did you, was it the traditional medical system as well as Allopathy, Ayurveda, Homeopathy, Physiotherapy etc. ?
6. Did the previous treatment provide you relief? Was there any recurrence?
7. Are you taking any medications or pain medication?
8. What is the intensity of the pain on the 1-10 scale?
9. What is the range of motion or the limitation in movement? (In the case of Musculoskeletal problems or discomfort).
10. Have you had any operation that has required modification of your body? (In the case of knee joints, joint implants,, or other procedures in which permanent modifications have been made to the inside)

It is possible to ask these questions and any questions you believe are pertinent. It is possible to inquire about Age when you're not in a position to make a judgment. But, I've never inquired about this particularly to women. I frequently ask people about their job and life style. This provides me with information on the type of mental or physical stress they experience or their postures when working. The people who use two-wheelers for a long time or use chairs for prolonged periods often experience back related issues.

I've found it is extremely beneficial to understand the background of the disease and how long it has affected and whether it's an acute or chronic illness. This has helped me greatly to build my knowledge base in the past 4 years, and also assisted me in selecting my treatment approach for the future. Today, I sense what I need to focus my attention and what method would be more effective. It also aids me in telling the person receiving treatment about what my experiences or experience with these ailments has been , and what they can expect.

In certain cases it can be helpful to check if the onset of the illness is linked to another event that occurs that has occurred in your life. individual. In many cases it is possible that a specific emotion might trigger the disease. Be aware that many illnesses are psychosomatic and have a psychosomatic cause. It is important to note that the time of the incident and the moment when the illness first manifests could not always be in sync because, often after the incident, it can take several months before the disease can manifest or get more severe. When a health issue appears and becomes serious it could have had an interval of 6 months to a year also.

Conducting a pre-assessment of the issue:

I suggest that prior to beginning the healing process the practitioner must perform an objective assessment of the severity of the condition i.e. the degree of discomfort, pain or restriction in motion range when it's an issue of the musculoskeletal type. Sometimes, I don't take this step because of insufficient time or because of the urgency of getting into the healing process.

In the pre-assessment, if there is any type of pain, you must seek an assessment of the severity of the pain using one-to-10 scale. 1 indicates very light 5 is considered average and 10 is severe. The score you get before beginning the healing process allows us determine later whether there's any effect, and If so, what the extent. Sometimes it is the case that the health issue or pain does not resolve entirely, even after a single session. In such cases it's important to be aware of how much improvement you can expect every session. In one case I recently treated I began the healing process with the initial level of pain being 8/10. After a 5-minute healing session, the pain level dropped to four on 10,, and it completely disappeared after the second treatment session that lasted 10 minutes.

If a person suffers from issues like an Frozen shoulder, prior to the session of healing it is a great suggestion to ask the patient to lift their hands in order to determine the range of motion achievable. If someone is experiencing knee pain Then request them to get up from an upright position and assess the level of pain and the level of discomfort standing. If constipation is the cause Ask them about the typical frequency they empty their bowels. If you find a person who has irregular menstrual cycles it is possible to ask them for specifics regarding the regularity of their menstrual cycle and duration, dates or times.

I also suggest that you conduct an examination at a set interval throughout recovery. If, for instance, I am treating a patient who is suffering from an injured shoulder, after approximately five minutes of healing, I usually request that they examine if there is any change in the level of pain or mobility.

The purpose of this session is to clarify what can be expected in the aftermath of your healing sessions:

Before your healing sessions, it's recommended to take a few minutes discussing the potential issues that the person participating in the healing session may experience after the session. It will help them understand what to be expecting.

I generally inform patients upfront the slight chance that no improvement occurs. I also remind clients they have a possibility that their health issue could temporary worsen, and their pain may get worse or shift to a new location as part of healing. I also inform them that, while the majority of patients get completely healed in one short appointment, there have been instances that require several sessions over a longer time.

I also inform them that ultimately, their body will decide how quickly healing can occur. I explain to them that the deeply rooted the issue is and how it affects how healing proceeds. I inform that chronic issues may be more difficult to resolve while acute issues may be resolved more quickly. Additionally, issues due to incorrect posture could be resolved quicker, but problems due to emotional reasons could be resolved only after the emotional problem is addressed. I also inform those who have successful in curing their condition and reverting back to the same way of life or posture they had before it will be a recurrence when it is time.

I once treated one of the drivers who worked by my client. He was suffering from severe painful foot pain on his left. He said that the pain was due to a hefty clutch in the vehicle which he was driving. Luckily , he was completely healed from pain during the healing process. I advised him that if he kept driving while using the hard shifter, pain could likely return in the next few weeks or even months.

Do's and Don'ts

1. Be sure to remain relaxed when you are doing your healing session. Your mental health as a healer is extremely crucial. If you're being stressed out or in a state of disorientation mind, avoid any healing sessions. Each of the methods I've mentioned require a calm and peaceful mind.

2. I suggest that if you can get into the state of zero points without difficulty, regardless of the technique you're employing, try to enter this state while you're healing. I have discovered that it to speed up the process and help heal extremely quickly.

3. It is a good idea to keep our mobile phones on silent and to request that the other person maintain their cellphone in silent mode.

4. When the healing process is ongoing, continue engaging with the person at regular intervals. Initially , I was thinking that this would keep me from focusing and take me away from the zero point. But, I realized that it helps me

stay aware of both, even when the healing process is going on.

5. Make sure to check their comfort regularly and ensure that you are also at ease during the workout.

6. Ask them to give you feedback every time they notice any changes within their body. This will give you an indication about where you'll need to focus your attention.

7. Simply keep your awareness within their body. They don't have be thinking of something, sing or even pray.

These tips must be considered before, or throughout the healing session. These points must be explained to the person prior to the session to ensure they take the necessary precautions prior to and during any healing sessions.

***

***

Chapter 14: T1 - Heart Energy Healing

This chapter introduces the healing technique that relies on Heart energy. The first portion of the chapter offers information and a step by procedure to perform the healing. The next section provides the personal experience of healing through this technique.

Part I: Technique

This technique utilizes the electro-magnetic energy of the heart to heal. This is nothing but the sensation of Love which we feel within our hearts. It is actually an Scalar energy form that can be transmitted in any direction , and across distances without losing strength or intensity. I've used this healing technique across distances as well. It's truly magical in nature.

In the past three years, I've tried my method for healing over 200 patients with remarkable results. A few of my experiences are nothing short of miracles. This healing method is easy to grasp and to apply. It is possible for anyone to begin practicing it within five minutes of having read this chapter. Before we dive into the process Here are some information regarding how to work with the Heart Chakra and Heart Energy.

Our Heart is an vital organ. While it may appear that pumping blood is the sole role that the heart has, it's believed that the heart actually functions as an endocrine gland that releases crucial hormones essential to live a healthy and happy life. At a spiritual level the heart chakra functions as an encirclement known to be the Anahat Chakra. The heart is about loving self and others, relationships and compassion, empathy and forgiveness. It is also about acceptance, acceptance, the ability to transform, change, to grieve and achieve peace, compassionate discernment centers of awareness as well as the integration of knowledge. The heart chakra when it is in a state of open it allows us to feel a deep interaction and harmonious exchange of energy that surrounds us, and we begin to appreciate all that is wonderful.

It is important to note that the Heart Chakra is not exactly the place where the Heart is however it is located in the heart's center. It's 4th Chakra which is also called the Energy Vortex starting from the Root Chakra. There are 7 Chakras which are energy vortices within our bodies. They exist in both energy and as physical form within the body. In the energy form, they are present as frequencies of specific frequencies that I have described in the next section. While in the physical, they are glands of endocrine ducts that are not ductless.

The Root Chakra i.e. the Mooladhara Chakra is associated with the Prostate , Testes, and Ovaries. The second Chakra above it corresponds to that of the Swadhishthan Chakra i.e. Adrenal Gland. 3rd Chakra Manipur Chakra i.e. Solar Plexus and represents the Pancreatic Gland. The fourth Chakra can be described as known as the Anahat Chakra i.e. Heart Chakra or Thymus Gland. The fifth Chakra is known as the Vishuddhi Chakra also known as the Throat Chakra i.e. Thyroid as well as Parathyroid Glands. The sixth Chakra is known as the Adnya Chakra i.e. the pituitary gland. The seventh Chakra is known as the crown chakra i.e. Pineal gland.

It is believed that the Heart chakra is located in the middle of the body, having 3 Chakras over and 3 below. It plays a crucial part in healing. I've observed that sending a light stream of white light energy of love to an area of the body that is affected immediately initiates healing.

The process is quite simple. It is beneficial to first open the heart chakra before I begin sending heal energy towards the person. In order to do this, I first shift my attention towards the chakra of the heart i.e. to the region right to the center of your chest(Not precisely where the heart is however it Is in the middle) . After that, I tap the chest gently with my fingers which assists in activating the chakra. It's also known as Thymus tapping. I perform this for approximately 30-40 times. It should be gentle tapping, and not something that can cause harm to us. At times , I simply tap my fingers three times on the area, then apply circular pressure to the area.

It almost immediately brings me an amazing feeling of warmth in my heart. After that, I take just a few minutes becoming aware and attentive to the sensations that occur in the heart area. I stay for about 2 minutes experiencing this feeling. After that, as I breathe in, I imagine energy coming into my body from outside and accumulating within the heart chakra area. Then I envision the energy expanding and becoming amplified. These easy steps aid in the building of energy within the Heart chakra and can be utilized to heal self or other people.

If we notice enough energy accumulation within the heart chakra, it is then time to transfer it to the body part that requires healing. Imagine a ray of light and love flowing through your heart chakra and onto the body of the other. To increase the intensity of love, consider any person who creates a strong sensation of love in your heart. This could include your child, parent brother or sister, puppies, kittens or any other animal that brings a sense of affection. When you inhale, turn your focus to the heart chakra. Then, every time you exhale continue to send heart energy to the body of the other. Repeat this process for about 5 to 7 minutes. It's as easy as that.

The fundamentals of this method are as follows:

A. A desire to heal
B. Awareness or consciousness of our body.
C. Deep Breathing - Exhalation and inhalation
D. A deep feeling of Love within the heart.
E. A Mind that's entirely silent and is not tied to the result.

Based on my experience, of these five fundamentals A, C and D are simple. A (i.e. the state of awareness) as well as E (i.e. the Silent Mind) are difficult for some. My observations are that if you can accomplish "B", then "E' i.e. the mind is usually silent. occur as a consequence from this consciousness.

Fortunately I was able to manage these issues after a few days of training.

Don't worry about how you'll achieve this. I'm certain you'll succeed particularly since my own experience of success in healing occurred during the very first clinical trial I conducted on a woman with back pain that was severe. I've mentioned this earlier in the chapter of this book. After just 5 seconds of treatments, she became totally healed. I'm sure you as well, on your first try, can achieve similar outcomes. This technique is very effective. Simply try it and be convinced.

Here's the step-by step procedure that you have to follow:

You should sit before the person you want to heal. Remember that you are not the one who is healing. The power of Love is performing this healing. you're just a conduit by which that love is accessible to the person who is being healed.

Step 1: Inhale the sensation of love in your heart. (Somewhere in the middle of your chest, next to the physical heart is your Heart Chakra /Vortex). Imagine it as if it's filled with a fervent love. If you're unable to feel the love within your heart, consider those you cherish deeply, like your child, father or spouse, mother and a puppy or kitten, etc. Simply feel the warmth of love in your heart area. It is helpful to me to push my shoulders a little behind and my chest slightly inward. It basically pushes the sternum up and produces a feeling of a heart that is more open and a greater sense of affection. You should try to feel a feeling of being one with and a heartfelt connection between you and your partner.

Step 2: Continue to breathe through and out regularly for 5-10 minutes. With each inhalation take your focus to your body, starting with your toes and moving up towards your head. Imagine how you would feel when someone was physically touching your body, sweeping their hands over your feet and moving until your knees, legs the chest, abdomen, and neck, and finally your head. As you exhale consider what you'd feel when someone touched you as they moved down from your head towards your shoulders and wrists and fingers.

As you breathe, you're conscious of the entire pathway from your feet up to your head when you exhale. Likewise, as you exhale you are conscious of the entire pathway from your head to the fingers on your hand. You must keep this state of mind through the entire healing procedure. Be aware that your breathing needs to be a little higher than the one we normally do typically. The ability to maintain these awareness-based sweeps is crucial. This will increase the energy of love that we built in our hearts during step 1. When you have completed step 2, you need to simply add step 3.

Step 3. Now, with the intention of healing each when you exhale, release an intense beam of heart energy to the area which needs to be healed. Each time you exhale and imagine a stream brilliant white or golden light coming from your heart towards the part that needs healing. Take a look at the area you are healing by using an eye that is focused. This helps focus your energy and focus on the correct spot. For instance, if you are helping someone suffering from painful knee joints, take a look at the joint, and when you exhale, channel the energy of affection towards the joint. Repeat this process for the next five minutes. Keep your body's awareness while you work. The body awareness can also assist you achieve a quiet state of Mind . It will also assist in increasing the heart's energy.

Step 4: As steps 1,2,3 is going on and you're sending the love of your heart into the physical body of your loved one, notice whether there is changes in his/her body. In essence, you should look for signs of healing. Find out if the person or she feels other than normal within. Most people experience an intense feeling or lightness, tingling sensations pins and needles burps and a cold or hot sensation or cold sensations, etc. Be aware of these since they are the signs that tell us that the shift is taking place within the.

At first, until you become accustomed to this method, try it only for five minutes. After that, take a break for 2 minutes, and then repeat the exercise repeatedly for 3-5 minutes or until you feel comfortable. Sometimes, people experience a feeling of hyperventilation when they breathe deeply. If this is happening to you, you should not take a deep breath. Instead, you should breathe normally, maintaining the rest of your procedure the same the way it was before.

I suggest that prior to you begin treatment, you first determine the degree of discomfort or pain on the scale of 1-10 (1=nothing five = average and 10= extreme). After the treatment, you should check whether there has been any changes in the degree of discomfort. Most of the time, you will observe a change. In the majority of cases, I've found that patients report a decrease in pain immediately or within the next day following an evening of relaxation for the body. In essence, the body requires an amount of time to allow all the Vata, Pitta, Kapha forces working together to take the disease from the system. The degree of relief depends on the individual's body's i.e. it's capacity to initiate healing and depends on the severity of the issue.

In the majority of cases, you will not require a repeat session because they are totally healed, but in the event that there is left-over pain after the session, you can repeat the session lasting 5-7 minutes the next day, using the exact same procedure. Keep in mind that awareness and Love are two main factors that are important.

It is crucial to be aware because it allows us to keep our energy at a high rate so that their energy and frequency rises to match ours and we don't have to go downwards to meet their frequency due to the effect of the entrainment. When you do this, ensure that your eyes remain fixed on the part of your body being treated. Concentrating our eyes aids in directing our attention towards the location we want to focus on. There is no need to worry whether we're in the correct place. I've noticed that energy efficiently goes to where it is most needed. Even if your focus isn't exactly in the right spot but it's not really a matter of to much.

This technique is a great option for remote healing at the distance. To do this, you'll have to take a picture of the individual or you'll have to create an icon of the body of the person. Send the intense affection to the photo or to the icon you've created or discovered.

Through this method I have noticed that our body utilizes the energy in a manner that is comfortable. I once treated someone with an injury to a finger using this technique. The on the following day, he told me that his finger felt improved, but what he discovered the most shocking was that the tooth that was painful for several days, had stopped hurting at night. Notice that I wasn't conscious of the pain in his tooth when I was undergoing his healing. We must realize how the human body can be smart enough to know where to apply the energy available.

Try this method and, believe me when I say there's no turning back. You'll be amazed by this easy and efficient method to heal. I have used it on animals, birds as well as insects, plants as well as other animals that are considered non-living.

This method can be utilized to treat ourselves too. It is possible to send energy of love to any body parts, or employ a mirror to channel the energy of love to the body part that is suffering. The energy to the power of Heart Energy is simply amazing and can surprise you every time I attempt this method.

Part II: The Healing Experience

Here's a case study of healing with the above method. This will provide you with an idea of how the procedure is carried out.

In December of 2016 I was in the capital city of Delhi to lead an educational course to Reliance General Insurance. In our tea break I spoke to the attendees about the healing I provide, and suggested that , if anyone was suffering from medical issues, I would assist them in a brief healing session. A person suffering from extreme neck pain came to me right away, and others took a break for an afternoon tea. Some decided to stay and see what kind of healing I would perform for him. I asked him specifics about the situation. He said it was difficult for him to rotate his neck sideways or to move his neck up and down with no suffering.

If I asked him to assess his pain on an 1-10 scale the answer was 8/10, which indicated for me that he experienced considerable discomfort. He informed me that he was going through the physiotherapy treatment for a number of months but didn't get much relief. Based on this basic knowledge, I set off with my healing procedure. I chose to utilize my Heart Energy Healing method which is described in this chapter.

I requested him to sit comfortably in a chair. I stood about a foot behind him to ensure the neck of his apparent to me. I informed him that I would perform the healing for 5 minutes and then we would check the degree of discomfort.

I also assured him that I will not touch him, and that he should only be able to hear my breathing out and in and out, nothing other than that. I instructed him to remain aware of his neck throughout the next 5 minutes.

I started to feel a sense of love within my heart. It was a strange day. I wasn't able to quickly trigger a powerful feeling of love within my heart chakra. I tried to imagine my little girl and all the ways I loved her. I imagined that I were hugging her with a tender hug. As quickly exactly as I had hoped I was able to feel the warm sensation of the love that was within my heart.

Then, I began breathing with a normal rhythm, however slightly deeper than my usual. As I breathed I focused my whole attention to the body. In the chapter above, I began moving my awareness from my toes towards my head. As I breathed out then I would shift my attention from my head to my fingers. Within a couple of seconds, I was conscious that my whole body was aware. Then I was able to bring my attention to the intense sensation of love that was forming in my heart. This feeling of love is what I now projected his neck to initiate healing.

Then I began the healing process. Inhaling and exhaling with a series of conscious movements I began to send powerful love beams towards his neck. I imagined that an intense beam of love and unconditional affection was coming from my heart towards his neck. I repeated this for 5 minutes, each time I would give him a number. Four minutes later, 3 minutes, 2 minutes, 1 minute just a few seconds until I finished.

Then I informed me that I was done with my process of healing as I asked him to see whether there had been any changes in the neck discomfort. The patient moved the head left and after which he moved it to right going up and down several times, then returned with a sense of awe. He informed me that his pain was completely disappeared. The neck was completely free which allowed him move his neck without feeling any discomfort.

Then, he inquired whether I held his neck in my hands for two hours after my healing was over. I responded in the negative and informed him that throughout the duration, I stood about a foot from him and didn't ever touch him. A few of the participants who were watching my healing session, listened to what I had stated. As I inquired about about what the sensation he was feeling and why he was asking me that question, he revealed something very interesting and intriguing. He said that he noticed a pair of hands gripping his neck from behind , and the hands then lifted his head and adjusted the bones of his neck one at a time. As the bones adjusted to the correct places and he felt lots of pressure under each bone segment being let go.

The two of us along with those who watched this were awestruck to listen to this. They could clearly see that I was not in touch with the patient's body, and how he was completely free of his condition within just five minutes.

The next day, I realized there was another factor at the helm and that someone or something else likely a greater force was in the background, at work, quietly doing whatever needed for resolving the issue. He was thrilled to discover that the intense pain suffered for months disappeared after only 5 minutes treatment. I was happy to have had the chance to experience this instant healing. This has given me a thorough knowledge that the healing powers of the scalar power of love.

I've used this method for healing hundreds of patients, and each time it's resulted in positive results. The results are almost like miracles for people who have experienced something like this at first. Insofar as I'm concerned, I'm astonished that it didn't work.

Chapter 15: Basic Techniques

For thousands of years, people have sought ways to quiet their minds and their minds. It was usually a result of seeking access to deeper levels, to union with nature or with higher sources. The majority of these efforts were extremely difficult and required strict discipline, usually in the span of many years.

Eckhart Tolle's greatest contribution was to show a totally different method or rather the way to bring back knowledge that was long forgotten. It was the method of observation. This idea was the basis for further techniques. Many of these techniques earned the name of a tune, and is of which some are protected by trademarks. It's nearly impossible to draw a precise distinction between the method and the method of operation of these methods, even though at least two trends were born out of these techniques such as quantum healing as well as matrix transforms.

Quantum Healing

In essence, the mental faculties of the human brain are a thing. In spite of its incredible possibilities and the amazing structure the mind can almost live its own existence. A growing number of people are not capable of utilizing this marvel of evolution to their own advantage. Instead, they are relegated to the side of the road in which they are being a part of what's taking place in the present. One of the most common examples is the destructive thoughts that can result in anger, frustration, and destructive behaviors. There is no one who wants to think about to think about these thoughts, but they always make their way into the spotlight. In extreme cases, massive psychological disorder could consequence. In our apparently so modern and advanced times, the prevalence of psychological disorders is growing to a alarmingly high degree. It's not an isolated issue. Health insurance companies today spend large sums of money in the treatment of mental problems. Additionally there is a alarming growth of people being unable to perform their job due to mental difficulties. Who isn't aware of the seemingly confused characters who walk around in the streets muttering and talking about themselves? While the majority of"normal" people "normal people" appear to behave similarly. They just carry on their monologues in a quiet manner, or they are able to listen, without being noticed from the outside to the same music which is their thoughts every day.

Over the course of hundreds of years, individuals from various cultures have come up with various methods to access the innermost layers of their minds. It includes, for instance, the practice of meditation (autoor auto) suggestions and a high demand on the human mind with a high concentration, or actions that run into contact with physical limitations and exert a subliminal effect. The majority of these techniques can be justified and provide a chance for achievement, if only for a brief period of time.

However, there are now superior, and certainly quicker methods. Innovative approaches are remarkable because of their ease of use. To illustrate this, it is crucial to pay tribute to that of Eckart Tolle. Instead of becoming a less or more helpless persona of the mind's activities the mind, or of striving to manage this "obstinate and unpredictable entity" He discovered an alternative. The method of the observer.

However, enough of the theory Let's get to the practical aspect. Before I begin, I'd like to make an important point. The methods in this guide are mostly passive strategies. This means that you can't choose the outcome you want. In fact, the more you desire certain outcomes and the more you want it, the more it's going to be hidden from you. That's why I recommend that you approach this task in a calm manner and with no expectations. It's already a method of "letting go" which will make accessibility much simpler for you.

Fundamental Technique 1. Watching Your Thoughts

Before reading any further take a second to pause. You can use the right side of your hand (left-handed readers use your left hand) and then bring your index finger toward center of the forehead. If you feel your skin touch then ask yourself this questions:

"Where does my next idea is coming from?"

You may be experiencing an extraordinary experience at the moment and can sense briefly a pause in the typical "murmuring about your mind". Perhaps for just a fraction of a moment, but it's usually present. If that's the case, then congratulations! You've accomplished something that would require decades of lives to accomplish: a peacefulness of their minds.

If you've not had the pleasure of experiencing this, there's no reason to feel frustrated or anger. It's just a matter of practice to achieve the same mistake. Be careful not to be too zealous and don't attempt to achieve success by imposing discipline or personal training. This isn't going to result in success. Try to approach it with a playful manner. Remember your childhood, perhaps how you once walked across a new meadow or an unexplored territory. You didn't know the things you would discover but your behaviour was characterised by curiosity that was childlike. With this attitude, you are able to begin the most interesting journey of your life exploring your mind and your own consciousness.

The next basic method is to gradually introduce you to the position as an observer.

Exercise Basic Technique 1. (Observing the thoughts of your mind)

1.) Relax in a comfortable setting and shut your eyes. Your spine and back must be in a straight posture. This is also true the case for your neck which must not bow to the front. Your feet should, with your feet not crossing, be placed flat across the ground. Your hands should be placed on your thighs, but without touching.

The ideal spot for this is a comfy and solid chair with no armrests. I do not suggest lying down as the capacity of your conscious mind is typically better when in a standing position. In addition, the likelihood of falling asleep significantly higher in a position that you lie on.

2.) Let your thoughts flow and go, without having an impact on them. You just have to observe what's happening. It doesn't matter if you think they're "good" thoughts or "bad" thinking. Simply observe what's happening. You can play the position as an observer. Do not try to control anything or wish for a particular result. Let go and let the thoughts flow and completely.

3.) Ask yourself this question:

"Where do I get my next idea is coming from?"

Following this question, just be aware of what is taking place. Don't force to do anything. At the beginning the windows that appear to be at an unending thought might be, not at all, but they will be. Be aware of what's taking place. Observe. After a few times, you'll observe that these windows grow more and more. Once you are aware that your thoughts are leading to an independent, automatic existence and you're no longer the character of an observer, you should you should ask yourself this question again.

It is beneficial to practice this workout at least a few times per day. Be careful not to create a strict schedule that has obligatory time slots. Try to keep it in a relaxing and fun way. A few short workouts every day are more beneficial than a few long ones.

It's ideal when you can get off for this exercise around three times per day for 5-10 minutes per time. If you work, you can incorporate the exercise with a five minute bathroom break with no difficulty. For a complete and effective exercise, it's beneficial to create a "countdown". Every cellphone or smart phone has this function typically in the same menu the alarm clock and stop watch. If you don't have this option then you can create a standard alarm clock or egg timer that rings within 5-10 minutes. If you don't own an alarm clock on be on hand, just do this and trust your intuition about time.

You'll probably notice that you've already slowed down with the simple method of observation in the second step. If not, it's not an issue. Don't try to force anything. or a comment that I do not say often enough.

At first, you'll discover that it may take just a few minutes before a shift in your perception occurs. Therefore, it's best to ensure that at the very least one exercise every day is approximately 10 minutes to allow you to see the change in detail. You can schedule 15 minutes of exercise, but there's no need to be overly ambitious and perform hours of exercise. Remember: doing more doesn't necessarily mean more.

To gain greater access to the position of the observer It is also possible to alter the subject. Here are some suggestions:

"What is my next idea be?"

"When do I expect to see my next idea?"

"Which color will my next thought be?"

"What do I think my next thought be like?"

There is no need to adhere to this lingo. It is your right to come up with your own ideas. There are no rules that are rigid and, as a rule there is no way to make a mistake. Every method that assists you to play the position of an observer is beneficial. It's how easy it is!

For a final conclusion, a few short explanations on the basis of this method. Human beings are typically exposed to the seemingly involuntary and uncontrollable actions of their minds. In addition, they frequently associate their entire self-image and self-image to a set set of expectations of role models. In a way that is very simple this image might be like this:

"My name's Thomas.
* I am male.
* I'm aged 34.
* I am American.
* I am employed as an administrator for one of the companies that insures.
* I enjoy playing soccer.
My closest acquaintances consist of Michael, Alexander and David.
* I love eating spaghetti and tomato sauce.
* Etc.
If you ask anyone, they is able to make a lot of similar statements about themselves. These statements could be true in some way, but you're significantly more than what can be described by these statements. This isn't about precision like, for example the precise definition of the mix of spices to make the purpose of making the best tomato sauce.

Your life and you are much more than you think. Additionally numerous people living in modern times have lost their sense of unity or have a tendency to distract themselves by the apparent benefits of our modern times. Television with 100 channels and amusement parks, malls, or various restaurants are useful and could keep a person entertained for a brief period. However, often this is associated with distracting. It is a distraction, or an absence from your connection with all living things. It is a profound unity that is in all living things. It is a connection with Nature and with the cycle of existence or, if you wish it, the connection with the God-given source.

Every time you step into the position of an observer you'll realize that you have beyond the our culture, traditional self-image, which is typically described in exemplary statements such as those above.

Chinese philosopher Laotse was aware that the most difficult journey starts at the beginning. This is why I am inviting you to take the first step. You've got nothing to risk. There aren't any negative adverse effects or like that. Maybe you'll be surprised in a the best way in what your life can change.

Try it!

Emotional Training

The transition from the initial base technique is fluid however, this type of emotional training is essentially more or less the "mother of all methods". If you're in the position of an observer, you'll realize that this usually comes to a very pleasant feeling. Your mind is at peace and you are aware that you are looking at your mind - like everything else - but in a totally different way in a flash. From a point of view of unity with something massive. Another advantage is that you're no longer just a passenger of your existence and instead, you assume the role of captain.

The feeling may differ and there isn't a specific "target-setting". Also, it's crucial not to force any action. Just take note and observe.

Exercise: Basic Technique 2 (Emotional Training):

1.) Begin by taking note of your thoughts using the basic technique 1.

2.) After a while, you'll notice that your thoughts have slowed down or completely slowed down.

3.) Be aware of this state of mind and observe the way you feel. You might feel a sense of calm and peace. Love, happiness, or feeling of elation are also possible. It could be a basic feeling of deep-felt peace but intense emotions like intensely felt joy or ecstasy can be experienced, too. Each of these emotions is superior or less than one or the other.

4.) If you are experiencing an enjoyable sensation, shift your attention to this sensation. Be sure you're simply observing. Do not try to force any action. Be aware of the different emotions using an unwavering calmness. Explore these feelings. Be aware of no of these feelings being more or worse than another.

3)Bathe in the sensation Enjoy the moment. Enjoy the sensation until it reaches its limits.

4.) If the boundaries of this feeling are expanding take it as a sign to go along with the expansion. Allow yourself to drift off in a calm way, surrounded by these pleasant emotions, wherever they might bring to. Be calm and connect with the feelings and not put any pressure on. Be the emotion.

*****

Attention: If you think that thoughts pop in the middle and then push their way to the forefront simply go back one step. Don't be upset. Be aware of you thoughts and thoughts in a peaceful manner until you are able to experience that pleasant feeling again. Turn your attention to the emotion and experience it through the perspective of the observer.

*****

Attention: Get rid of any expectations. The feelings that are rising may be different. Sometimes, they are more intense and at other times, they are not so clearly perceived. Additionally, it may vary over time or over the course of an entire day, in the location and how you feel the emotions. Whatever way you experience the pleasant feeling It's a good feeling.

*****

Attention: Perhaps, for a short time you are unable to perceive any thing. In this case, you're in a state of pure consciousness, a state of not thinking. Don't worry about it, just take it in and enjoy it. Somewhere you will be able to see thoughts which you can see or you will feel the wonderful sensation over and over once more. Concentrate your attention on the feeling. Be aware of the quality and the depth of your emotion by observing it in a calm and yet mindful manner.

*****

Attention: It's quite easy. Whatever happens within your head you are just an observer. Imagine that you are in the theater and watching an upcoming film. Do not interrupt your thoughts or emotions. Never attempt to exercise any type control.

*****

To do this, you must be taking a few minutes each throughout the day. You can do it to start your day or take it up in the evening before bed, while you're to sleep. Additionally, this workout is perfect for letting the tension and stress that you have experienced throughout the day, and relax and drift off to sleep.

If you regularly practice these two fundamental methods can have already had significant effects on your daily life. You'll see that you're more peaceful and you've been able to get things in order with your self. Additionally, these exercises result in you to become more "authentic" due to your increased access to the innermost parts of who you are. Most often, your relationships with others improve and you can make better choices. Furthermore positive health effects are normal and you'll probably experience more restful and better sleep. Possible side effects: none. You are safe, and can't harm yourself by performing these exercises.

To help you with this exercise, there are a few additional suggestions that will gradually allow you to attain this higher state of consciousness to your everyday routine.

Addition Basic Technique 2 Transfer to everyday life I:

1.) After you've completed fundamental technique 2 Begin to slowly open your eyes.

2.) Try, using eyes wide to be aware of the sensation you felt. Feel that sensation with your eyes open.

3.) Between, you can close your eyes for two minutes in order to be in a position to be able to see more clearly what's taking place on the monitor of your brain. If you feel that the sensation changes then observe the new sensation without bias.

4) Open your eyes. Practice this mental training. Thoughts will come up as feelings and a state of pure consciousness, being able to not think.

5.) Try to gain access to your emotions again. Once you've regained that access, slowly get up. Be calm and steady with no jerky movements. Take a look at something near you and be aware of your feelings as you do that.

*****

Attention: The emotions could intensify, weaken or alter. However, this isn't any change in the sensation or its degree of intensity. They are more the various types of you which go beyond the self-concept with its anxieties and demands.

*****

The more you become accustomed to this likely new situation, the more will feel at peace with your body. You'll begin to view the world from a different viewpoint. Not only that, but this sense of unity and richness is the most ideal foundation for any possible change to your own personal situations. It's the ideal condition to build an all-new world for yourself.

As you can see, it's the intention to translate the state of being in harmony with the real you or your source of your being step by step into your daily routine. The following step will help you take one step closer to the goal. At first, you should allow approximately 15 minutes where you won't be interrupted. After some time , you'll be more comfortable with the method and you can decrease this time with no problems.

Addition 2: Basic Technique Transition to everyday life II:

1.) Do the fundamental technique 2 in the same way as you normally do until you feel a great feeling affirms that you've discovered your authentic self.

2.) Continue to remain in this state for five minutes or so.

3.) Then you'll slowly move one the fingers. Then, you can reconnect to the sensation you felt for five to 10 seconds.

4.) Then take a moment to move your fingers or even your entire hand until it is right for you. After that, you can return to the feeling repeatedly for 5 to 10 seconds.

5) Repeat the exercise with different areas that comprise your body. It is crucial to return to your sensation for 5 to 10 seconds afterward. The sequence is not important. For instance, you could start with your forearm followed by your upper arm, and at the end , the entire shoulder. Then you can move on to the arm and hand. You can also shift your gaze across your face from the nose, and the other way is to move from right eye towards your legs. It doesn't matter so long as you can consciously return to your sensation for a few seconds afterward.

6.) Then, focus in your thoughts for up to three minutes in order to finish the exercise.

The more time you spend in connecting with yourself and the awareness of the positive feelings that go along to it, the easier it will be to integrate this state of mind into your life routine and allow it to be "normal". In the next article, we will provide some suggestions on this subject.

Training Basic Technique 2 in Daily Life
Make every chance to connect to your authentic self. At first, take frequent breaks of between 10 and 60 seconds to reconnect with yourself. When you work, you are able to be glued at your computer screen. Utilize every opportunity to wait whether in the car when you're stopped at a red light or while you travel on public transport or in the photocopier at the office. Stop for a few minutes in the course of daily activities, such as cooking coffee or waiting on water to heat up or similar that allow you to feel familiar emotions.

Be aware of these feelings when you are doing tasks that are not demanding at the beginning. This could be as simple as making the table while brushing your teeth, or even doing your housework.

Gradually become aware of your feelings during the more intense activities.

If thoughts, particularly repetitive, automatic thought patterns are present, keep a routine of watching them, as if you were an animal perched on the mouse hole.

If you are successful you've achieved something that people have dreamed of for a long time. You're at peace with your own mind and are in control of your thoughts without stress. Additionally, you're connected to your real self, which is more than the typical small roles that society assigns to us.

Chapter 16: Synchronizing

Quantum physics is the method by which quantum physics comes into play that has changed the way we view our world. The scientifically verified and reproducible understanding that the expectations of the person carrying the experiment could affect the results of the experiment is a crucial factor. If you are tempted to believe that it's nonsense then you must search for "double-slit study". There are not only similar descriptions on sites with obscure content, but also on many pages with top-quality scientific orientation.

This revolutionary insight has led to more conclusions that everything is linked to everything. The conventional perspective of the world as a linear time as well as the at present, believed to be unchanging, relationship between cause and effect has been flipped upside-down.

In a sense, this is about the scientific proof of connecting powers. It was like a reversal. remote healing psychic experiences, telepathic experience and other strange occurrences weren't just bizarre nonsense any more. The quantum theories provided a framework of explanations for this phenomenon for the first time.

In reality quantum physicists aren't a the esoterics of the abyss. Quantum physics' results were considered to be so revolutionary and important in the sense that German scientist Max Planck was awarded the Nobel Prize in Physics for it in 1918. Since then, quantum physics theories have been further refined through numerous research studies which is why every book store will have a book regarding quantum physics in their selection of books.

If everything is somehow linked to each other, it will have a practical application for the people. The various methods of synchronization have two factors.

Aspect 1. Every living thing in the universe strives in spite of the apparent chaos to maintain a certain level of consistency and order. Particularly, nature is eager to find an equilibrium. One good example is the chaotic solar orbits, also known as planets and stars, which generally tend to be level in fixed directions and assist in "keep everything in place". When we look at our animal world, we observe that there is the tendency to have an optimal balance between the ratio of predators to prey. If the balance is at risk of becoming a mess The birth rate of either of these genera instantly changes. Additionally, new species may emerge or even disappear until a certain balance has been restored.

The more frequently and more specific an order is achieved by synchronization more beneficial for each element.

Two-way perspective: We prefer to judge facts that are objectively neutral. "Sickness is negative" and "health is good" is a simple illustration of this. Synchronization seeks to connect the oscillation range of undesirable conditions with the frequency of oscillation of the conditions that are targeted and thus increasing the overall frequency of oscillations.

In order to reach the point of synchronization there are many ways.

Exercise The Body Parts of the Body Synchronize

1.) Place yourself in an upright and comfortably on a seat as you did during the previous two fundamental methods.

2.) If you're right-handed, be aware of your left hand (left-handers their left hand). Simply observe your hand. Do not try to force anything, and don't change the way you feel. Take note, from your hand's position how it feels to lie in your thigh. If your hand is numb then it's good. If your hand is like it's tingling, that's great. If your hand feels warm or cold and feels warm, that's great in the way it feels. Even if you initially feel like you're not feeling anything It's fine. Observe. Then shift your attention towards your right hand.

In contrast to relaxation achieved through self-hypnosis or other methods like this, it is not a manipulative intent (heavy hand warm hand, heavy hand, etc.). It is only about the observation from the position of the observer. After a few repetitions, keep doing this until you can see something with your hand. To increase the accessibility and improve your ability to perceive hold your hand in your mind for around an hour afterward.

3.) Switch your attention to the other foot. Begin to feel your foot. Feel how your foot is touching the floor. Check the sole. Check whether your feet feel trapped by a sock, or a shoe. Consider how your feet feel. It is sufficient if your foot feels "somehow different" in comparison to your hand. When you notice this, stay in your foot , with your awareness and perception for around one minute.

4.) Switch again to your hands until can clearly see it. Keep your hands in place for approximately 1 minute.

5.) Concentrate your attention on the opposite hand of your foot again and stay there, with having a clear vision for around an hour.

6.) Switch between hand and foot approximately two to three times more, until the distinctions in perception get more obvious. You will eventually be capable of recognizing that your feet and hands feel different.

7) We are now at the actual sync. Combining the sensations of foot and hand in your brain. The feelings will move towards one to the point that they overlap and merge. Be aware of the sensation of hand and foot becoming one. Notice and feel. Stay in this state for a short time.

In the beginning , it's possible that your perception of the foot and hand is tiny. However, as you get more practice, you'll be able to see and feel more particulars.

*****

Attention Pay attention: This exercise isn't about imagining every tiny hair on your body and every pores. If you've trained your awareness of your body's organs a few times, it will be more and more possible for you. But don't create the mistake of making it a contest as it's the aim to experience more precise and different sensations each time. Enjoy your role as an observer. In the event that your senses become more precise and distinct after a time that is a good thing. If you notice your foot and hand more clear than you did the last time that is fine also. The purpose of this exercise is to detect distinctions in the conscious perception of body parts and the subsequent melting, or more accurately, the fusion of these two distinct sensations.

*****

Applications

As we build on the basics exercises, we are at the point of doing these exercises. Utilizing the two fundamental methods - the observing of your thoughts and emotional training, you will most likely benefit by a regular practice. You will see that your automatic thought patterns are losing their power, and that you're no longer the lone victim of the destructive loops of thoughts. Instead, you can take the steering wheel of your mind and mind to your own with regular education. This means that you become an active participant in your life and of your circumstances.

The applications are a lot more varied in the fundamental technique of the synchronization. But we can't consider the process of synchronization as completely autonomous because it is necessary to be in a state of emotional heightened for it, because it triggers through the first two fundamental methods.

Synchronization can be used in an effective way to heal many different issues. The most interesting thing is that it does not just perform well during self-application. Healing support for others or living beings is feasible. It is not necessary to be present. It is effective from a distance too.

To show the ease of using quantum healing, here's an illustration. You'd like to treat anyone who is suffering from tension or pain in his shoulder.

Training: Quantum Healing (e.g. shoulder):

1) Find out where they would put the intensity of the pain, ranging between one (barely visible) up to 10 (heavy and nearly unbearable pain).

2.) To avoid distraction to minimize distraction, walk to the side of someone. This isn't a must and is especially important when you don't have any practical experience and eye contact could appear to be a threatening interruption for both parties.

3.) 3. Place the tips of your fingers of one hand over the site or in the location where the pain was found.

(You could also utilize the entire fingertips or the entire hand. Use it in the method that feels the most comfortable to you.)

4.) Feel the area using your fingers as wide as is possible. Be aware of the surrounding area as well as the layers below.

5.) Look for an area that is pain-free using one hand. Be gentle as you move your fingers over that body part of the person you are talking to and be amazed at the direction you are taking your focus.

6.) Change once or twice back and to and using your conscious until you can feel the sensations.

7) Connect the emotions of the two spots. Feel the emotions that the spots merging into one. It could be beneficial to imagine the way the "pull" the sensations of the spot without pain towards the area that is painful through

your mind. After that, you should be aware of how these two sensations relate.

8.) Feel this feeling of connection for a time. Keep the state in mind and experience the feeling of being connected.

9) You can ask the person what the person would put the severity of the pain between 1 and 10.

Usually , the severity of the pain is less evident now. However, it could be a long time before the effects begin to take effect. It's not an issue. Do not try to force any thing.

Variations in the application

The principle is the same. It doesn't not matter if you choose to put this technique to use on others such as animals, yourself, or even from the distance. One of the advantages of this method is that any application you make on other people is beneficial to you too. What could be more beneficial? The more you help others then the more you take care of yourself. This is an ideal "win-win-situation" in the way that business studies tend to promote it.

Let's look at different ways of working. When working with others, you don't have to interact with them. It's enough to follow the steps within your mind. Let your intuition guide you. That's why this process is effective at a distance too. Do you think this is an absurd? You should test it out and see by what will occur...

Another option, which could help make quantum healing process easier for those of you who are suffering, is the recourse to an intermediary. This could be a pet or plant, a water bottle, or simply an image that you have in your mind. Apply the methods discussed above to this alternative. If there's no way to classify the pain that you're treating and you are unable to do so, then it is time to let it go. I will repeat my own words That you can't commit a crime and not cause harm.

Exercises to follow
In addition to the basic exercises, which were previously described there are a variety of other exercises that offer the benefit of. But,

a rigorous repetition of the basic exercises should never be overlooked. You may be able of accelerating your progress through more exercises since you are able to approach the center of your being by examining different aspects through these exercises. In addition, you may discover certain exercises so engaging or fascinating that you'd be interested in putting them to work. In this article, I'll provide some techniques that will help you in your journey.

www.ingramcontent.com/pod-product-compliance
Lightning Source LLC
Chambersburg PA
CBHW050408120526
44590CB00015B/1880